REMEDIATION CASE STUDIES

HELPING STRUGGLING
MEDICAL LEARNERS

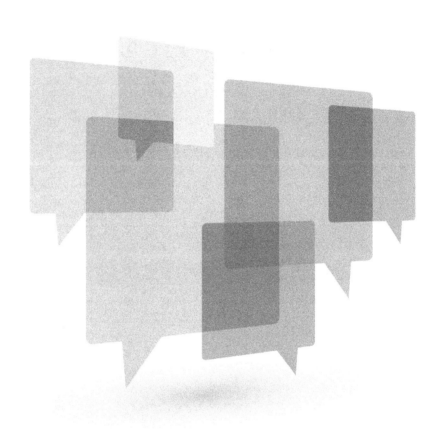

REMEDIATION CASE STUDIES
HELPING STRUGGLING MEDICAL LEARNERS

Jeannette Guerrasio, MD

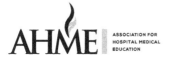

AHME | ASSOCIATION FOR
HOSPITAL MEDICAL
EDUCATION

The information in this book is presented in the form of cases with commentaries. The case examples are amalgams of real cases in which names and all identifying information have been changed. The book is based on information reasonably believed to be accurate at the time it was written. These materials do not constitute legal or related advice, and the reader should consider the contents of the book as providing general guidelines which will need to be individualized. Since the circumstances of each case are different and because it remains the responsibility of the user to retain the services of their own legal and/or other advisors when appropriate, neither the editor nor the publisher shall be held liable for the application of these guidelines. Based on cases submitted by multiple contributors, Dr. Guerrasio organized and prepared comments for this book. While these comments may coincide with the views of the Association for Hospital Medical Education (AHME), they are not a statement of AHME's policies and practices.

Association for Hospital Medical Education
109 Brush Creek Road
Irwin, PA 15642
724-864-7321   phone
724-864-6153   fax
info@ahme.org   email
www.ahme.org

The text of this book is set in Minion
Book designed by Michael Sayre

Printed in United States of America
1 3 5 7 9 10 8 6 4 2

Remediation Case Studies: Helping Struggling Medical Learners / Edited by Jeanette Guerrasio, MD

Library of Congress Control Number: 2021921406

ISBN 978-0-578-31063-3

Cover design by Michael Sayre

CONTENTS

ACKNOWLEDGEMENTS

Having worked together on multiple projects, including the books *Remediation of the Struggling Medical Learner, Editions 1* and *2* and *Guide to Medical Education in the Teaching Hospital*, this book marks yet another wonderful collaboration between the Association for Hospital Medical Education (AHME), its executive director Kimball Mohn, MD, and literary agent Joan Parker of Parker Literary Agency, LLC. I thank AHME for their assistance, encouragement, and championing of medical education. I've never been so impressed by an organization as I am with AHME and the dedication of its leadership and members. Thank you to Kim for his ongoing contributions and support; I only wish our paths would cross more often so that I could glean more wisdom and kindness from his presence. I give credit to Joan for her vision in suggesting that we put together a case studies book and thank her for her openness to my creative ideas, even at the most rudimentary phases.

This book would never have come to fruition without the generous time and offerings of our contributors (see list of contributors to follow). It was their dedication to medical education and to teaching struggling learners that provided the experience needed to add thoughtful cases, with helpful examples of remediation and insightful reflections. It should be noted that several of the cases presented in this book are conglomerates of more than one case. Some of the submitted cases were rewritten to achieve a consistent format throughout the text. Prior to publication, contributors were not asked to respond to editorial commentary, partly because that process may have resulted in an extensive loop: contributors' cases → editor's comments → contributors' feedback on editor's comments → editor's feedback on contributors' comments, etc.

For this book, my comments are meant to offer constructive advice and useful criticism; my intention is to be helpful. Overall, we trust that readers as well as contributors will understand that my goal is to advance medical education for the sake of improving patient safety.

Reflecting on my experience in the field, I am thankful for every individual and institution that has welcomed me onto their campus to learn and to share ideas. Everything that I have learned from you has been, in some form, packaged and incorporated into this book as well.

I also wish to thank the mentors who have encouraged my professional development in this field. First and foremost is my primary mentor Eva Aagaard, MD, who is remarkably talented in every domain of medical education. Thank you also to my first and most effective remediation team: the late Maureen Garrity, PhD, Terri Blevins, EdD, and Carol Lay, EdD. I miss you every Wednesday and all the days in between. Thank you to others who have helped lead me and shared in this journey: Carol Rumack, MD, Suzanne Brandenburg, MD, Steve Zweck-Bronner, JD, Rebecca Maldonado, PA-C, Ethan Cumbler, MD, and Juan Lessing, MD. Thank you to Adina Kalet, MD, Calvin Chou, MD, Carmella Nogar, PA-C, and Karen Warburton, MD, for being colleagues and continuing to carry this work forward.

Thank you to Lara Juliusson, my pillar of strength at home, who supported me as I dared to write two books simultaneously while caring for a full internal medicine practice – during a pandemic.

CONTRIBUTORS

Virginia Adesola Adewole, MD
Faculty
Los Angeles County / University of Southern California Medical Center

Paula Algranati, MD, FAAP
Clinical Associate Professor
Bay Path University Physician Assistant Program
Professor of Pediatrics (retired)
University of Connecticut School of Medicine

Nikolai Butki, DO, MPH, FACEP, FACOEP
Residency Program Director of Emergency Medicine
McLaren Oakland Hospital, Pontiac, MI
Associate Professor, Osteopathic Medical Specialties
Michigan State University College of Osteopathic Medicine

Rachel Byrne, MS, PA-C
Clinical Faculty
University of Colorado School of Medicine Child Health Associate/Physician
Assistant Program

Dominique Cosco, MD, FACP
Associate Professor of Medicine
Residency Program Director of Internal Medicine
Washington University School of Medicine

Steven R. Craig, MD, MACP
Adjunct Clinical Professor of Medicine
Assistant Dean (Des Moines Branch Campus)
University of Iowa Carver College of Medicine

Kelsey Dougherty, MMSc, PA-C
Assistant Professor
University of Colorado School of Medicine Child Health Associate/Physician
Assistant Program

Daniel B. Frank, MD, FACEP
Assistant Professor, Zucker/Hofstra School of Medicine
Residency Program Director of Emergency Medicine
South Shore University Hospital / Northwell Health, Bayshore, NY

Lisa Hearns, MPH, C-TAGME
Graduate Medical Education Manager
Pine Rest Christian Mental Health Services
Michigan State University

Kylie Horne, MBBS, FRACP, PhD
Director of Clinical Training, Monash Doctors Education and Consultant in
Infectious Diseases
Monash Health
Senior Lecturer, Faculty of Medicine, Nursing and Health Sciences
Monash University, Melbourne, Australia

Christina Johnson, MBChB, FRACP, PhD
Director, Monash Doctors Education and Consultant in General and Geriatric
Medicine, Monash Health
Adjunct Clinical Associate Professor, Faculty of Medicine, Nursing and Health
Sciences, Monash University, Melbourne, Australia

Janita Keating, BAgrSc, PGDipEd, PGCertProjMn, DipTraining&Design
Monash Doctors Education Manager
Monash Doctors Education
Monash Health, Melbourne, Australia

Tamsin Levy, MD
Associate Program Director
Highland Hospital, Oakland, CA

Wendy Lim MBBS, FACEM, GCCT
Director of Clinical Teaching, Monash Doctors Education
Emergency Physician, Dandenong Hospital
Monash Health, Melbourne, Australia

Lawrence K. Loo, MD
Associate Dean for Faculty Development
Chauncey L. Smith Professor of Medicine
Loma Linda University School of Medicine
Loma Linda, CA

Andrew Mastanduono, MD
Associate Residency Program Director for Emergency Medicine Residency
South Shore University Hospital - Northwell Health
Assistant Professor of Emergency Medicine
The Zucker School of Medicine at Hofstra University/Northwell Heath

Susan McDiarmid, MS, PA-C
Assistant Professor
Director of Clinical Education
Bay Path University Physician Assistant Program, Longmeadow, MA

Cristina Nituica, MD
General Surgery Residency Program Director
Central Michigan University College of Medicine

Carmella Nogar, PA-C
Instructional Faculty
University of New Mexico

Andrew S. Parsons, MD, MPH
Assistant Professor of Medicine and Public Health
Associate Program Director, Internal Medicine
Director, Clinical Reasoning Coaching
Director of Pre-Clerkship Coaching and Clinical Skills
University of Virginia School of Medicine

Bill Sanders, DO, MS
Psychiatry Residency Program Director
Pine Rest Christian Mental Health Services
Michigan State University

Jacqueline Sivahop EdD, PA-C
Associate Professor, Associate Program Director
Child Health Associate/Physician Assistant Program
University of Colorado School of Medicine

Archana Sridhar, MD, M.Ed
Assistant Professor
University of California San Francisco, San Francisco V.A. Medical Center

Amy Steinway, OD, FAAO
Assistant Clinical Professor
State University of New York College of Optometry

Indhu Subramanian, MD
Associate Clinical Professor
University of California San Francisco
Program Director
Highland Hospital, Oakland, CA

Chad Vercio, MD
Chair Department of Pediatrics
Riverside University Health Systems Medical Center
Assistant Professor of Medicine
Loma Linda University School of Medicine

Deborah Virant-Young, PharmD, BCPS
Director of Faculty Development
Michigan State University College of Osteopathic Medicine
Statewide Campus System

Mary Jo Wagner, MD
Designated Institutional Official
Professor, Emergency Medicine
Central Michigan University College of Medicine

Karen M. Warburton, MD, FASN, FACP
Associate Professor of Medicine
Director, Clinician Wellness Program
Director, GME Advancement
University of Virginia School of Medicine

Lijia Xie, MD, MS
Faculty
Highland Hospital, Oakland, CA

Introduction

N OW IS THE perfect time to introduce a book of case studies to the blossoming field of medical learner remediation. In its infancy only 15 years ago, the field has produced a growing list of literature and even a few books on how to help struggling medical learners. The works include evidence-based and eminence-based tips on how to approach the struggling learner with new methods of early identification of underperformance, suggestions on how to best understand a learner's deficits, how to triage the educational needs of a struggling learner, how to build and implement efficient and effectual remediation plans, how to find appropriate resources, manage institutional legal concerns, address changes to each learner's academic status, and ensure competent graduates. What we don't know yet is how these newly discovered techniques and practices are being implemented in the field and whether or not they work across various institutions and learning environments. A look into cases studies from around the world is one place to start. It gives us a window into what has worked and not worked in the remediation of struggling learners.

In 2006, I had just completed residency and was a first-year internal medicine attending at the University of Colorado School of Medicine. To everyone's shock, the internal medicine program residency hadn't filled – the only year that happened prior or since. After much debate and programmatic self-reflection, we easily identified that the residency program had a new program director, an interim chair of the medicine department, and had announced that the hospital and medical school would be relocating to a new campus. Instability was perhaps not a successful selling feature.

After "The Match," in which fourth-year medical students are paired with their future residency programs, our internal medicine program had filled over 50 positions, yet had 5 vacant seats remaining. The medical students who ended up backfilling these openings were students who had submitted their applications and interviewed at other residency programs but had not been accepted. Most of these medical students were not even planning on going into the field of internal medicine, but neurology or psychiatry instead. As a result, 4 of the 5 learners hadn't completed a general medicine rotation in well over a year.

Within weeks of the intern class's arrival that July, it became clear that there was a large performance gap between the 50-plus students who had been accepted through The Match and the 5 students who had come through the backfill process known then as "The Scramble" (now called "The SOAP," which stands for Supplemental Offer and Acceptance Program). With time, the gap only widened. Each day, the 50-plus students were learning avidly from everything around them, while the 5 students seem to move around unknowingly, their education flying uncaptured over their heads.

With my love for teaching, seemingly unlimited patience, and a direct communication style, I can only guess that these are the reasons I was asked to help bring these 5 students up to speed with their peers. In the process, I was tasked with building a remediation program for the Internal Medicine Residency Program. With great enthusiasm I accepted the role with what I thought was a fail-safe plan. I would go to the library and read every article there was to read about how to remediate struggling residents and what was needed to build a remediation program. Then I would reproduce what I had learned at my home institution.

Don't you love the naïveté and eagerness of young faculty? In my first literature search, I found a few papers describing the struggles of residents and medical students who had fallen behind. There was an internal medicine survey of program directors in 2000 that quantified the prevalence of internal medicine residents in need of remediation, what the most common identified deficits were, how they were identified and by whom.[1] At the time it was the most comprehensive research study on struggling learners.

In 1998, there had been a study of 144 anesthesiology residency training programs, inquiring about remediation policies, probation, and the appeals process.[2] Each study represented only one program at a single institution. The topics of these rare studies were limited to remediation policies, remediation of in-training exam scores, and descriptions of struggling residents. There was no reliable data or instruction on how to remediate struggling learners or how to build a successful remediation program.

My next step was to call program directors who had been in their roles for years and had worked with struggling residents. Through our conversations I learned that the standard remediation plan of the time was (a) letting the learner know what they needed to improve upon, (b) assigning the resident a mentor who gave general or vague advice, (c) having them repeat rotations, and (d) providing them with a deadline to demonstrate improvement.[3] That was the "what" part of the process, but I wanted to know the "how." How did the residents go about improving? The response was often along the lines of, "We just hope that by having more exposure to patients they will learn what they need to know," or, "Sometimes I watch residents graduate and honestly, I am a bit unsettled that they will be taking care of patients. I hope they know when to ask for help." Ultimately, what I learned was that almost all the remediation programs consisted of having the struggling learner do more of the exact same things that they had been unsuccessfully doing in the past.[4] Albert Einstein has been credited for saying, "The definition of insanity is doing the same thing over and over again but expecting different results." Now, I don't think these program directors were insane, nor the learners. They just didn't know what else to do and didn't have the time or resources to figure it out.

I have spent the rest of my academic career trying to get to the big question, "How?" After working with the first cohort of learners, I wrote a book called *Remediation of the Struggling Medical Learner*[5] which I was able to publish and distribute thanks to the Association for Hospital Medical Education (AHME). We eventually updated that version with a second edition[6] after I had worked with hundreds of learners and had accumulated more experience. The books were meant to gather everything that I had read and learned though my own experience, and through the experience of others along the way, into one place so that the hypotheses and practices could be more rigorously tested and studied at multiple medical centers. I also wanted the techniques to be tested across levels of learners from students to residents, fellows and attendings, and across disciplines from nurse practitioners to physician assistants, physical and occupational therapists, pharmacists to optometrists. At the University of Colorado, we have had tremendous success using nearly identical techniques across all stages of learning, medical specialties, and various medical disciplines.

In *Remediation of the Struggling Medical Learner*, I outline an approach for remediation that begins with methods for identifying struggling learners as early as possible, knowing that early identification and intervention are associated with improved education outcomes.[7] Once the struggling learner is identified, a differential diagnosis of their educational deficits is determined from the following list of possibilities which was expanded from the original Accreditation Council for Graduate Medical Education (ACGME) competencies.[8]

- Medical Knowledge
- Clinical Skills
- Clinical Reasoning
- Time Management and Organization
- Professionalism
- Communication
- Interpersonal Skills
- Problem Based Learning and Improvement
- Systems Based Practice
- Mental Well-Being

Mental well-being is defined as any stressor that the learner brings into the learning environment that affects their ability to learn, such as depression, substance abuse, learning disorder, birth of a child, sick parent, etc. The same framework will be used throughout this text.

Most struggling learners have multiple deficits, and the strategy is to pick the greatest deficit and build a remediation plan to tackle that one deficit.[9] For example, if a learner struggles with clinical reasoning as their main deficit, they often collect too much information during a patient encounter and write longer notes, not knowing what is important. This presents as a time management problem. When presenting, they will have trouble communicating a plan, since they often struggle to make one. This leads to the learner also being identified as having a communication problem. Because the learner is having trouble making quick decisions, the nurses begin going over the learner's head to ask others for patient orders. Noticing this, the resident begins to struggle with self-esteem and depression.

If we can fix this learner's clinical reasoning, the other deficits will magically go away. Once the underlying deficit is isolated from all other deficits, remediation plans are designed around K. Anders Ericsson's work on deliberate practice, focusing on practice, receiving direct actionable feedback, followed by reflection and an opportunity to practice new skills in a cyclic model.[10]

Since 2006, the research on remediation of the struggling medical learner has expanded to include other great texts such as *Remediation in Medical Education*[11] and *Learning from Lapses: How to identify, classify and respond to unprofessional behaviour in medical students.*[12] Original research studies and commentaries on the subject have multiplied exponentially, adding both evidence and breadth to our understanding of the subject. Now it is time to see what others have implemented around the United States and the world. Have others found success with the remediation of their learners? Are the published remediation techniques working beyond the institutions where they were studied and first implemented? Are there remediation strategies being used that have not yet been formally published? What can we learn from studying examples across different disciplines and levels of learners?

While I was originally asked to help 5 residents, I never lost sight of the greater mission which was to ensure patient safety and to make sure that every patient who interacts with a clinician gets reliable, trustworthy, satisfactory care. This is why I quickly expanded my program to include medical students, residents, and fellows from all specialties, and attendings and students of other medical disciplines.

Having now worked with over 800 learners and hundreds of individual training programs, it comes as no surprise that I frequently run into former learners. Their gratitude feels great, but I am most amazed by the comments that reflect evolving insights from the work we did together and how they use what they learned mindfully in daily practice.

What I didn't anticipate was the degree to which engaging in this work would change me. It has made me a more observant teacher of all learners, a better teacher overall, a more articulate and thoughtful provider of feedback, a more self-reflective clinician in my own practice and in other aspects of my professional career, more compassionate towards learners who experience the world differently, more informed of the complexities of the evaluative process, and more appreciative of the roles of the deans and program directors.

It is difficult for patients to truly know if their provider is practicing evidence based, standard of care medicine. We have the privilege of being a self-regulated profession. With noble aspirations, I take that charge very seriously. We have an ethical obligation to invest our time, resources, and energy in remediating the deficits of our colleagues and soon-to-be colleagues for the sake of our profession and all the patients that literally put their trust in our hands.

I put a call out for remediation cases through my publisher, AHME, and contacted experts in the field requesting their input. The cases have all been deidentified, edited, and combined when similar. The submitted cases and contributor names have been separated to further conceal the identity of the referenced individuals. Please see the list of contributors to appreciate their efforts and recognize the diversity of contributions.

As you move through the cases presented, you will see that they have been generously contributed by faculty from MD, DO, PA, and OD schools and include cases involving struggling students, residents, and attendings. While I did not receive any cases from nurse practitioner schools or physical therapy schools this time, remediation efforts have been successful there as well.[13]

The cases included were edited for consistency of presentation and clarity. *My comments appear in italics.* Some may wish to read the text cover to cover, others may prefer to choose cases based on the challenges that they address. For that reason, I have included after each case number the learner deficits that were identified by the contributors. The deficits listed may not always match the case as it is presented. This may be due to variations in how learner challenges are categorized (since some of the competencies overlap), conscious or subconscious attempts to avoid particular labels, or because we are receiving only abridged summaries of individual cases. Giving the contributors the benefit of the doubt, I will presume that it is because we only have part of the cases, but will comment accordingly. There are times that I point out what could have been done differently. This is not meant to be critical, and it is quite possible that the remediation efforts included my suggestions in their plan but not in their case description. My suggestions may not have been possible either, and by the way, is there an easier position than being the Monday morning quarterback? My comments are purely meant to highlight key remediation points and common errors that lead to failed remediation.

There is a wealth of knowledge in the following cases. Enjoy learning from your colleagues in our vast global medical community. ⌨

REFERENCES

1   Yao DC, Wright SM. National survey of internal medicine residency program directors regarding problem residents. *JAMA*. 2000 Sep 6;284(9):1099-104.

2   Rosenblatt MA, Schartel SA. The problem resident-Probation and remediation in American anesthesiology training programs. *Anesthesia & Analgesia*. 1998 Feb 1;86(2S):180S.

3   Cleland JA, Milne A, Sinclair HK, Lee AJ. Predicting performance cohort study: is performance on early assessments predictive of later undergraduate grades? *Med Educ*. 2008;42:676-83.

4   Audétat MC, Laurin S, Dory V. Remediation for struggling learners: putting an end to 'more of the same.' *Med Educ*. 2013 Mar;47(3):230-1.

5   Guerrasio J. *Remediation of the Struggling Medical Learner*. Irwin, PA: Association for Hospital Medical Education; 2013.

6   Guerrasio J. *Remediation of the Struggling Medical Learner. 2nd Ed*. Irwin, PA: Association for Hospital Medical Education; 2017.

7   Denison AR, Currie AE, Laing MR, Heys SD. Good for them or good for us? The role of academic guidance interviews. *Med Educ*. 2006;40(12):1188-91.

8   Carraccio C, Wolfsthal SD, Englander R, Ferentz K, Martin C. Shifting paradigms: from Flexner to competencies. *Acad Med*. 2002 May 1;77(5):361-7.

9   Guerrasio J, Garrity MJ, Aagaard EM. Learner deficits and academic outcomes of medical students, residents, fellows, and attending physicians referred to a remediation program, 2006–2012. *Acad Med*. 2014;89:352-8.

10   Ericsson KA, Krampe RT, Tesch-Römer C. The role of deliberate practice in the acquisition of expert performance. *Psychological Review*. 1993 Jul;100(3):363.

11   Kalet A, Chou CL. *Remediation in Medical Education*. New York: Springer; 2014.

12   Mak-Van der Vossen M. *Learning from Lapses: How to identify, classify and respond to unprofessional behaviour in medical students*. Amsterdam: Gildeprint; 2019.

13   Horton C, Polek C, Hardie TL. The relationship between enhanced remediation and NCLEX success. *Teach and Learn Nurs*. 2012 Oct;7(4):146-151.

REMEDIATION CASE STUDIES

HELPING STRUGGLING
MEDICAL LEARNERS

CASE 1

Medical Knowledge, Clinical Reasoning, Time Management and Organization, Communication, Interpersonal Skills, and Mental Well-Being

LEARNER AT TIME OF IDENTIFICATION FOR REMEDIATION

Georgia, a second-year physician assistant student

REASON FOR REMEDIATION

The university's physician assistant (PA) curriculum consists of a 12-month didactic curriculum followed by clinical curriculum for another 12 months. Georgia had completed her first year of PA school and was promoted. However, she was quickly identified as a struggling learner when she started her clinical rotations early in her second academic year. After receiving information from her clinical preceptors that she was underperforming, Georgia was referred by the Director of Clinical Education to the remediation team. This occurred during her inpatient internal medicine clinical rotation, the second of 11 four-week scheduled clinical rotations.

> *Editor: Although Georgia may not have realized it at this point, she was very lucky for two reasons. First, while being identified as a struggling learner so early in her clinical rotations may have knocked her confidence, she had*

faculty that cared enough about her to get her help right away, when she still had over nine months to improve her skills. Early identification improves the chances of remediation success.[1,2] Secondly, she was lucky that her PA program had a remediation team with experience and faculty with expertise,[3] as such faculty are more successful at remediating struggling learners.[4] This type of team was able to put their minds and experiences together to analyze her challenges, identify her deficits, and create and implement a remediation plan with a high likelihood of success.

The remediation team was informed that she was at risk of failing the clinical rotation but for the time being was performing at a level of "low-pass." The goal was to utilize early intervention in hopes of improving Georgia's performance to a passing grade.

Georgia's clinical preceptors listed the following issues for the remediation team to address:

- A poor foundation of medical knowledge
- A lack of engagement in the rotation (e.g., not asking enough/ appropriate questions)
- Poor documentation skills; taking too long to complete notes, and her notes "weren't good enough"
- Not receiving feedback well; "defensive and a bit confrontational"
- Not completing chart reviews before going in to evaluate patients
- Did not appear to be researching topics that were assigned to her

More specifically, the remediation team found that Georgia was anxious about asking questions. She was rewriting her notes at night to improve upon them. Because she was occupied with rewriting notes, she was unable to do a lot of reading. She was embarrassed regarding the feedback as it was provided to her in front of the other medical learners and team members. She did not know how to review charts in the manner the team was expecting. She did research topics but got very anxious when asked to present to attending physicians. She stated that she felt very self-conscious. Additionally, she was internalizing the feedback, taking it personally and having a difficult time receiving criticism.

Editor: There are so many benefits to having a remediation team available to collect more information. Rarely is any one event an isolated issue that can be addressed quickly. The team can identify and clarify all the deficits that need to be addressed and search for specific examples of those deficits. In this case, it is unclear what about Georgia's notes isn't "good enough" and how they need to be fixed. The team can also detect patterns of behavior and gauge the severity of the learner's issues based on their experience with working with other learners.[5,6,7] *The team can also verify what the preceptor is seeing and ensure that the learner is being treated fairly and without bias.*[8] *Legally it protects the institution from a learner complaining about one particular preceptor treating them unfairly.*

In the introduction, mental well-being was defined as any stressor that the learner brings into the learning environment that affects their ability to learn. Certainly, in this case, Georgia's anxiety seems to overlap with perfectionism, at least when it comes to writing notes. This is a common challenge for struggling learners, many of whom are Type A personalities. It also can be very difficult for students who so desperately want to be perfect, and have been so successful in the past, to receive corrective feedback.

In addition, struggling learners are often unaware of the expectations for their performance. In this case, Georgia may have been too anxious and distracted to have heard the expectations when they were presented. At other times, expectations are not provided in a direct manner. Instead, faculty expect learners to pick up on the hidden curriculum and intuit what is expected of them. The hidden curriculum refers to the unwritten lessons, values, and perspective that learners gather while in training.[9] *Struggling learners usually miss the hidden curriculum. It just isn't how their brains are wired. They need to be told explicitly what is expected from them.*

REMEDIATION APPROACH

The remediation team hypothesized that there were several issues presenting concurrently. There were obvious time management and organization strategies for managing patient care that Georgia hadn't learned or been taught. In addition, the remediation team believed that she was mismanaging time by rewriting notes at home rather than reading and learning about her patients and their medical conditions. Time spent on her notes was contributing to deficits in medical knowledge and clinical reasoning. Furthermore, the remediation team concluded that some of the procedural difficulties were contributing to her anxiety about competence and overall performance. The team alleged that if Georgia's time management and organizational skills improved, her presentation skills and communication of medical knowledge would subsequently improve. Finally, the remediation team also wondered about the possibility of prior issues with anxiety.

> *Editor: The remediation team wondered whether she had prior issues with anxiety. Why didn't they ask? Faculty are not allowed and should not diagnose their learners; struggling learners are not their patients. But they can observe, "You appear anxious." Anxious is not a diagnosis. Let the learner respond, then ask, "Has this happened before?" "What have you tried doing to make yourself feel better when this has happened in the past?" If that approach makes you uncomfortable, ask about some specific behavior. "I noticed that you rewrite your notes. Why do you do that? Did you do that in college?" "Did you try anything to help with that feeling that caused you to keep rewriting papers in college?" Perhaps when she moved to PA school, the learner lost access to her provider and just needs your help with a referral. If asked the right questions, learners can reveal a lot of information that can be used to help them.*

After the initial meeting, the following plan was discussed and agreed upon with Georgia:

1. She would meet with the lead preceptor the following day and review the remediation team's discussion and plan.
2. Georgia would communicate that she understood her identified deficits and would proceed forward with the following plan:
   a. She will read at night and no longer rewrite notes at home; rather she will spend her study time reading about 1-3 topics regarding patient care per night.
   b. She will record brief summary notes (from her reading) on index cards so that when presenting to attending physicians, she will feel less anxious.
   c. She will check in with her preceptor on a regular basis to see how things are going, at a minimum of once a week.

d. She now understands how and why to review patient charts prior to evaluating the patient.

> *Editor: It may also be helpful to tell a learner to write their notes in bullet points or sentence fragments rather than full sentences. Students who seek perfection are then less likely to get caught up in grammar and punctuation, saving countless hours.*

At a first follow-up meeting three weeks later, Georgia told the remediation team that her initial meeting with the lead preceptor went extremely well, as did subsequent check-ins. She received feedback that initial week, and then the next week, that her notes and overall performance were much improved. She still had residual fears (she was "very anxious") about "writing a bad note."

> *Editor: Frequent in-time feedback is so important and, as in this case, can help reframe expectations around note writing. I suspect that Georgia's expectations were still different from her preceptors.[10] For example, feedback will help her know whether she needs to be making changes to how she writes her notes and if this attending or rotation has similar expectations as the last.*

After the first follow-up meeting, the remediation team encouraged Georgia to continue actively seeking feedback, reading at night rather than rewriting notes, and reviewing patient charts in advance. Additionally, the remediation team suggested that Georgia seek help at the university counseling center to combat her anxieties regarding poor performance. Georgia was in complete agreement with the plan.

The remediation team continued to meet with Georgia in person approximately once a month for five to six more months. Over the course of the first few months, they identified additional mental health issues.

Early on, Georgia had revealed to the remediation team that she "wanted to jump out of the window because she was so mortified by her performance." The remediation team explored the concern of potential suicide risk at length and ultimately were convinced that she was not in any imminent danger. "Oh no, I like myself too much to do this to me or my family; it's just an expression to convey how mortified I felt." They did refer her back to counseling and kept in close contact with her; she did not repeat any similar statements.

Editor: Student and resident suicide is a reality that we must consider and address.[11] Our learners in remediation are at heightened risk because they are under more pressure, experience higher levels of scrutiny, and aren't getting the daily rewards that their peers are experiencing – despite the fact that they are working as hard, if not harder. Inquiring about suicide risk is the correct thing to do as well as making the appropriate referrals. Don't hesitate to call police for a welfare check, call an ambulance, or walk a learner down to the emergency department.

On a deeper dive into Georgia's past faculty encounters, it was learned that during her second semester of the didactic curriculum, her academic advisor referred her for counseling due to anxiety and to the university's academic success center for time management concerns. Georgia did not proceed forward with the academic advisor's recommendation for counseling services because, although she admitted she was anxious, she didn't feel she had the time needed to make an appointment and actually engage in the counseling process. She did, however, meet with the university's academic success center once to discuss time management skills and study techniques. This speaks to the initial identification of mental well-being and time management concerns during the first year of the PA curriculum.

Editor: And herein lie many challenges. Learners cannot be forced by an institution into treatment, and student privacy concerns prevented subsequent educators from knowing that previous challenges had been identified but inadequately addressed. Perhaps there could have been better follow-up of this learner from the counseling center or the academic success center. The importance of feeding information forward will be addressed in several subsequent cases (see Cases 5 and 19). Many students and residents also need help finding protected time for provider visits for mental health counseling and prescription monitoring.[12] This is something educators can proactively offer.

In exploring mental health issues further, Georgia later told the remediation team that she had been mauled by a dog when she was younger, an incident she described as a traumatic experience. Georgia explained she went to counseling for several months following that incident. At the time, counseling had been a very positive and reassuring experience for her. This gave her very positive feelings about mental health counseling, thus leading her to be open and accepting about the remediation team's subsequent referral for counseling.

Over the course of several follow-up meetings, Georgia ultimately revealed that during the inpatient internal medicine rotation, another medical learner (a PA student from another institution) had actively sabotaged her during the workups of some of the patients. This other medical learner had been at the rotation for several weeks prior to the start of Georgia's rotation. Georgia had been reluctant to inform the remediation team earlier of these details and refused to include this information in her written feedback about the clinical site and preceptors. The remediation team assured Georgia that this feedback would be provided to the appropriate faculty involved. It is believed that this, too, was a contributing factor towards the performance anxiety that Georgia experienced, especially in the first few weeks of the rotation.

The team's overall strategy for remediation was to allow Georgia to air her own concerns (letting her tell her story) while conveying to her what her preceptors' concerns were (they told their story). The team served as coaches who guided her to problem solve and develop strategies to overcome hurdles and identify deficiencies. A non-judgmental and non-pejorative approach allowed Georgia to open up to the remediation team. This process revealed prior uncontrolled mental health issues, some of which may have been ongoing and contributing to her anxiety in the clinical rotation setting. The team assured Georgia that they were her advocates but also maintained high performance standards and expectations.

Two faculty members (one full time and one adjunct with extensive remediation experience) met with Georgia during the 6 months of remediation for the first half of her clinical year. An experienced mental health professional met with her in consultation on several occasions during this same period.

DISCIPLINARY ACTION

No disciplinary actions were taken or necessary in this case. With the early intervention of the remediation team, Georgia was able to improve her performance and decrease her anxiety. She ultimately earned a grade of "pass" on her preceptor evaluation of clinical competency for the clinical rotation.

HINDSIGHT REFLECTIONS FROM THE TEAM

In hindsight, one thing the remediation team might have done differently was to obtain a more thorough mental health history at the initial meeting and/or seek more information from Georgia's academic advisor. We believe this would have unveiled her prior issues around anxiety. This could have led to a very early mental health referral and perhaps a more collaborative remediation plan. A second consideration is that it may have been prudent for Georgia's academic faculty advisor to follow up with her regarding the counseling referral during the didactic year.

However, having said that, this case highlights the balance that must exist between PA faculty and their students. Per accreditation standards, PA faculty must be educators and not medical or psychiatric clinicians. Referrals can be made for medical and psychiatric interventions, but we must remember we remain in our educator roles as PA faculty.

> *Editor: If you send a learner for an evaluation, please include a physical and psychiatric evaluation. As wisely mentioned above, you are not their clinician. If you refer only for a psychiatric evaluation, you may find yourself in the middle of an unwanted lawsuit for having presumed a diagnosis. I learned this pearl of advice from program directors across the United States in a variety of training programs and across disciplines, many of whom didn't have access to an organization like a Physician Health Program that provides comprehensive evaluations. Consider sending the learner to both a primary care doctor and a psychiatrist or psychologist (see Case 17).*

Finally, this case reveals the importance of early intervention in the remediation process of a struggling learner in conjunction with open communication of all faculty (including clinical preceptors). The initial communication between the clinical preceptor and the director of clinical education regarding the clinical preceptor's concerns allowed for an early referral to the remediation team. Ultimately, this led to clinical rotation success for Georgia. She passed the remainder of her clinical rotations and the board examination on the first attempt. ⌕

REFERENCES

1 Denison AR, Currie AE, Laing MR, Heys SD. Good for them or good for us? The role of academic guidance interviews. *Med Educ.* 2006;40(12):1188-91.

2 Winston KA, van der Vleuten CP, Scherpbier AJ. Prediction and prevention of failure: An early intervention to assist at-risk medical students. *Med Teach.* 2014 Jan 1;36(1):25-31.

3 Winston KA, van der Vleuten CP, Scherpbier AJ. The role of the teacher in remediating at risk medical students. *Med Teach.* 2013; 34:e732-42.

4 Winston KA, van der Vleuten CP, Scherpbier AJ. Remediation of at-risk medical students: theory in action. *BMC Med Educ.* 2013;13:132.

5 Chou CL, Kalet A, Costa MJ, et al. Guidelines: The dos, don'ts and don't knows of remediation in medical education. *Perspect Med Educ.* 2019;8:322-338.

6 Cleland J, Leggett H, Sandars J, Costa MJ, Patel R, Moffat M. The remediation challenge: theoretical and methodological insights from a systematic review. *Med Educ.* 2013;47:242-51.

7 Mattick K, Knight L. High-quality learning: harder to achieve than we think? *Med Educ.* 2007;41:638-44.

8 Toretsky C, Mutha S, Coffman J. Breaking barriers for underrepresented minorities in the health professions. Retrieved from Healthforce Center at UCSF website https://healthforce.ucsf.edu/publications/breaking-barriers-underrepresented-minorities-health-professions. 2018 Jul.

9 Hafferty FW. Beyond curriculum reform: confronting medicine's hidden curriculum. *Acad Med.* 1998 Apr 1;73(4):403-7.

10 Hewson MG, Little ML. Giving feedback in medical education: verification of recommended techniques. *JGIM.* 1998;13(2):111-6.

11 Hampton T. Experts address risk of physician suicide. *JAMA.* 2005;294(10):1189-91.

12 Campbell S, Delva D. Physician do not heal thyself. Survey of personal health practices among medical residents. *Canad Fam Phys.* 2003;49(9):1121-7.

CASE 2

Communication and Interpersonal Skills

LEARNER AT TIME OF IDENTIFICATION FOR REMEDIATION

William, a third-year physician assistant student

REASON FOR REMEDIATION

William failed his emergency medicine rotation. Despite having very good medical knowledge, he was failing at interpersonal skills with both patients and his preceptor. His patients experienced him as off-putting, which was attributed to his flat affect. They commented that they felt like he wasn't interested in them. The patients stated that they did not believe he was a nice person and had not listened well enough to gain an understanding of their situation. At his worst, he would laugh inappropriately, including when a patient was being given bad news.

William had a perceived "negative attitude" that did not endear him to his preceptors or the rest of the emergency department staff. He made preceptors feel like he did not want to be there and was not interested in learning. They felt his affect, laughter, lack of empathy, and inability to connect with patients were enough of a professionalism issue that he should not pass that month's rotation.

Editor: Such behaviors can present under numerous circumstances. First, it will be important to determine whether he has the requisite skills and is choosing not to use them, or if he doesn't have the skills. Does William have autism and struggle with social skills? If he has the skills, is there a reason that he isn't using them? Is it arrogance? Perhaps he already knows that he wants to go into surgery and feels that this rotation is unimportant or beneath him. This tends to be a bigger problem on primary care and psychiatry rotations. Is his reaction an attempt to hide poor clinical reasoning? More investigation into the diagnosis of his educational deficits may be warranted to look for other deficits and to see if he has the needed skills but is not using them in this environment.[1]

REMEDIATION APPROACH

When William initially failed his emergency medicine rotation, he was discussed in the physician assistant promotion's committee meeting. It was determined that he needed remediation to address his poor interpersonal skills. He was put on probation but allowed to continue his rotations, as the committee felt he could best work on his deficits while on a clinical rotation. A team of 3 faculty members was identified to create and implement the remediation plan.

Following is the list of remediation tools utilized (in approximate chronological order):

1. A meeting every 2 weeks with a member of the remediation team (team members took turns). The meetings were tailored to the point William was in the process and included a review of his deficits, discussion of his assignments, brainstorming alternative behaviors, reviewing site visits, etc.
2. A review of prior video-recorded simulated patient exams to identify areas of weakness and ways to improve.

   Editor: This is most effective if the learner is asked to role play new techniques or actually repeat the simulated patient scenarios. Talking alone doesn't allow for mental incorporation of the new techniques. He must deliberately and actively practice the skills.[2]

3. Reading an article about the importance of effective communication in healthcare and writing an essay reflecting on how this is important in his case.

Editor: Essays are great, as are any form of active learning. Remember, professional identity formation is a gradual process of maturation.[3] It is hard to resist making corrections to another person's essays or thought processes, but learners must progress on their own timelines. Trying to force development doesn't work and only creates rifts and conflict between the teacher and the learner. Just let the learner reflect where they currently are in the maturation process. Remember, learners don't need to have insight to begin remediation or to change their behaviors.

4. Since the remediation team could not find an evaluation document that pertained specifically to William's deficits, they created one. (See **Appendix A**) The remediation team reviewed and discussed this document with the student.

Editor: This document sets expectations and is clear and concise. It is a wonderful tool that can be used as is or adapted to individual learners and their specific challenges.

5. One of the remediators and a faculty clinical coordinator performed site visits while William was on his next 2 rotations. Using the form that was developed, the remediators observed the learner and his interactions with coworkers as well as patients.
6. The remediators met with William to review the site visits and what they observed, including the comments on the communication form.
7. At the simulation center, 3 standardized patient exams were specifically tailored to the learner's deficits.
8. William was required to comply with the plan his remediation team created, pass subsequent rotations, retake his ED rotation, and have the promotions committee agree to remove him from probation.

William was extremely receptive to every aspect of the remediation. By the time of his first site visit, his interpersonal behavior was already much improved. For example, he was actively showing empathy with other providers and patients. He was smiling (instead of having a flat affect) and showing positive body language towards patients. He did well on his simulated patient exams and received good marks from his subsequent preceptors. Finally, he passed his repeat emergency medicine rotation.

DISCIPLINARY ACTION

After initially failing his emergency medicine rotation, William was put on probation. Requirements for successfully completing remediation were met, including passing the rotation that he had failed, and he was taken off probation.

SUCCESSES

The team felt that it was most successful at identifying specific deficits and targeting those in building their remediation plan for the student. The most effective strategy was providing real-time feedback based on the remediation team's direct observation of the student's interactions – both with patients and their families in clinic, and with simulation patients. The team-based approach helped spread out the workload.

OPPORTUNITIES TO LEARN

The team initially had no idea how to run a remediation. Of the three of them, two faculty and their remediation coordinator, only one had been involved in a case – and it was related to medical knowledge. They felt as though they were making it up as they went along. There was confusion among program leadership as to what actions were allowed as part of the remediation (ex: does doing a site visit violate FERPA? *No*). The team actually met with someone from the legal department to get guidance. There was almost complete lack of historical information of how the program had run remediation in the past. The single document from a prior remediation was not helpful, as it was geared towards aiding learners with medical knowledge deficits.

> *Editor: Kudos to the group of faculty for doing something that was new and for finding success. This is an encouragement to readers who may encounter similar challenges and not find success easily. Clearly, what was done here worked! Remember, there are common patterns that exist across learners, and general remediation plans can be used with learners that have similar challenges. At the same time, each individual is unique, so some aspects of general templates may need to be individualized.*[4,5,6]

Seeking legal counsel is always a wise idea and should be done early. Ideally, the lawyers will have experience and encourage you to do the right thing for patient safety and for the learner. Their role is to provide you with backup and protect the institution. Not all legal teams have experience and are familiar with legal precedent in this area. Work with them so as not to escalate anxiety or create extra work, but rather to ensure that you are following your institutional policies.

Documentation need not be voluminous, but it does need to be clear, concise, accurate, and timely. Remember that documentation serves many purposes: to help (if possible) convince the learner that they have a deficiency, to guide the remediation plan, to justify grades and disciplinary actions, to protect individuals and institutions from legal action, and to guide future remediation. It also gives you a chance to establish what works and what doesn't work at your institution.[7]

HINDSIGHT REFLECTIONS FROM THE REMEDIATING FACULTY

Looking back, we are actually very impressed with what we put together, not having done it before. The steps we took to teach William were specific. He was able to work on specific communication skills and did very well. In hindsight, it would have been nice to have had a plan for how this was to work. Trying to create it ourselves was stressful and time consuming.

> *Editor: There are some resources in the literature, but certainly more evidence-based research in this area is needed.*
> - *Regan L, et al. Remediation methods for milestones related to interpersonal and communication skills and professionalism. JGME 2016;2(1):18-23.*
> - *Guerrasio J. Remediation of the Struggling Medical Learner Ed 2. Irwin, PA: Association for Hospital Medical Education; 2017.*
> - *Guerrasio J, Aagaard EM. Long-term outcomes of a simulation-based remediation for residents and faculty with unprofessional behavior. JGIM. 2018 Dec;10(6):693.*

REFERENCES

1 Guerrasio J. *Remediation of the Struggling Medical Learner, 2nd Ed.* Irwin, PA: Association for Hospital Medical Education; 2017.

2 Ericsson KA, Krampe RT, Tesch-Römer C. The role of deliberate practice in the acquisition of expert performance. *Psych Review.* 1993 Jul;100(3):363.

3 Cruess RL, Cruess SR, Boudreau JD, Snell L, Steinert Y. Reframing medical education to support professional identity formation. *Acad Med.* 2014 Nov 1;89(11):1446-51.

4 Chou CL, Kalet A, Costa MJ, et al. Guidelines: The dos, don'ts and don't knows of remediation in medical education. *Perspect Med Educ.* 2019;8:322-338.

5 Bearman M, Molloy E, Ajjawi R, Keating J. 'Is there a Plan B?': clinical educators supporting under-performing students in practice settings. *Teach High Educ.* 2013;18:531-44.

6 Yellin PB. Learning differences and medical education. In: Kalet A, Chou CL, editors. *Remediation in Medical Education: A mid-course correction.* New York: Springer;2014.

7 Guerrasio J. "The Prognosis is poor:" When to give up. In: Kalet A, Chou CL, editors. *Remediation in Medical Education: A mid-course correction.* New York: Springer;2014.

CASE 3

Communication and Professionalism

LEARNER AT TIME OF IDENTIFICATION FOR REMEDIATION

Joe, a second post-graduate year resident in internal medicine

REASON FOR REMEDIATION

In May, Dr. Joe, a second post-graduate year internal medicine resident on his night float rotation, was paged by a nurse named Yoruba. Yoruba was caring for a patient with known heart failure. There was a standing order to give this patient 80mg of intravenous furosemide. The patient was hypotensive, and the nurse contacted the cross-cover resident, Dr. Joe, to discuss her concerns about giving this diuretic medication to a patient with low blood pressure. Dr. Joe communicated to Yoruba that his calculated mean arterial pressure (MAP) was different than her reported MAP. According to Yoruba, Dr. Joe became confrontational and rude. Yoruba was so upset that she then paged the internal medicine attending physician to discuss the concern and situation. In addition, she reported Dr. Joe to the head of nursing in a formal complaint.

Additional background was provided for context, as follows. Dr. Joe is a resident who is originally from Lebanon and who completed medical school in Beirut before coming to the US for residency training. The nurse is originally from Nigeria. Dr. Joe had had complaints about his communication style previously. The prior complaints, from earlier the same year, reported that his tone was inappropriate and there was a perception that he "orders" around his female resident colleagues.

Editor: It is not uncommon for residents who have been referred to remediation to cite that they were referred because of a singular incident, while the faculty or program director can recount several events or an identified pattern of concerning behavior.[1,2] Struggling learners are notoriously poor self-assessors.[3,4] Even though no comment was included as to any conversation or intervention that may have followed the first reported complaint, it sounds like an educational moment may have been missed to provide Joe feedback about how he was being perceived, intentionally or not. It could have been an opportunity for growth and understanding, even if the resident was unjustly targeted due to bias. Regardless of the cause, if it happened once, it will surely happen again, either in residency or beyond.

REMEDIATION APPROACH

Remediation occurred over the next 3-4 months, directed by the chair of the remediation committee and the resident's associate program director. The approach to this case was as follows:

1. In a meeting with his APD, Joe was asked to recount the night's events with Yoruba. His recollection was congruent with what nursing had reported. The APD asked Joe to reflect on why the nurse perceived his communication as confrontational and rude. The focus of the conversation was designed to help him gain insight into how he is being perceived by other members of his team (nursing, peers).

   Editor: Thankfully, the details of the case were agreed upon and there was not a battle of he said versus she said. If such disagreements arise, quickly bypass the details of what was said, as they are not the problem. The problem here is the non-verbal communication, the style of communication, and the perception of his communication, not the content. That should be the focus of attention.

2. The APD asked Joe to reflect on his communication style for the next 2 weeks and try to identify areas or times when his intent did not match the perception of others.

Editor: Sometimes learners need prompts, such as, "Consider not just the content of what you said, but also your tone, your volume, the pace of your speech, your posture, your choice of words, whether you think the listener felt heard, etc."[5] Most residents lack such self-awareness and are better served by having a trusted team member to help point out when their actions may not be well perceived. This can be done after an interaction through verbal feedback or in the moment through an agreed-upon sign or signal, like a hand gesture or phrase.

3. To their surprise, the resident came back to his APD with insightful reflections that stemmed from a discussion he had with his wife. She had given him insights into how others perceive him and his communication. He was able to process the feedback with his wife. They were also able to identify cultural differences with communication styles that he found enlightening and interesting.

4. The APD then facilitated a discussion between Joe and a female resident peer to discuss his communication and what worked and did not work. She gave very direct feedback and examples from when they worked together.

   Editor: Not every program will have a colleague who is so generous as to provide such difficult feedback. What a gift!

5. Joe made a plan for future inpatient rotations to set communication expectations with his team on the first day. He shared his goals with the team and attending, telling them to let him know if his style was becoming too authoritarian.

   Editor: Struggling learners who hide their deficits, hoping to fly under the radar until graduation, always fare the worst. They feel alone, isolated from their peers, and often become targeted by frustrated and angry colleagues. On the other hand, struggling learners that are transparent about their challenges enlist the help of their peers, who by nature are driven to help others, to create teams of support and encouragement... most of the time.

No further communication issues were brought to the residency program or documented on evaluations for this resident's third and final year of residency.

DISCIPLINARY ACTION

No disciplinary action was given due to the engagement level of the resident in the remediation process.

SUCCESSES

The self-reflection piece was very helpful, but the two interventions that worked the best were: (a) the resident talking to trusted individuals (i.e., his wife) about the perception that he was "ordering" others, and (b) the facilitated discussions with his peer in a safe sharing space.

HINDSIGHT REFLECTIONS FROM THE REMEDIATING FACULTY

We should have addressed the communication issues, specifically tone, immediately when the issues were raised by his peer residents. ⏎

REFERENCES

1   Chou CL, Kalet A, Costa MJ, et al. Guidelines: The dos, don'ts and don't knows of remediation in medical education. *Perspect Med Educ*. 2019;8:322-338.

2   Guerrasio J, Aagaard EM. Long-term outcomes of a simulation-based remediation for residents and faculty with unprofessional behavior. *JGME*. 2018 Dec;10(6):693-7.

3   Patel R, Tarrant C, Bonas S, Yates J, Sandars J. The struggling student: a thematic analysis from the self-regulated learning perspective. *Med Educ*. 2015;49:417-26.

4   Hodges B, Regehr G, Martin D. Difficulties in recognizing one's own incompetence: novice physicians who are unskilled and unaware of it. *Acad Med*. 2001 Oct 1;76(10):S87-9.

5   Beebe SA, Beebe SJ, Redmond MV. *Interpersonal Communication*. Scarborough, Ont.: Prentice-Hall Canada; 2000.

CASE 4

Professionalism, Communication, and Interpersonal Skills

■ LEARNER AT TIME OF IDENTIFICATION FOR REMEDIATION

Pat, a first post-graduate year general surgery resident

■ REASON FOR REMEDIATION

Shortly after Pat's matriculation into the general surgery residency, the program leadership received several concerning comments and complaints about him. Nurses and midlevel providers described him as rude and disrespectful, showing little deference or respect for the experience of veteran nurses and midlevel providers. Supervising attending physicians similarly found Pat to be argumentative and disrespectful, especially in the presence of other staff – and even patients. Specifically, while he was representing the program on an outside rotation, he consulted an attending pulmonologist by phone and began raising his voice in anger and making derogatory comments after an apparent disagreement. The pulmonologist filed a formal complaint with the site director.

> *Editor: This is an unusual presentation. Individuals typically struggle with people they perceive to be either above or below them in the chain of command. To have challenges with both is less common. If a struggling learner only*

has challenges in one direction, then you can confirm that they have the necessary skills, but just need to employ them more broadly. In this case, we don't know whether he has the necessary skill set.

The program leadership also learned of several social media posts made by Pat that drew concern. In one particular post, Pat lamented missing an opportunity to see a patient who required a thoracotomy. The post simply mentioned the procedure without noting any concern for the well-being of the person involved. Pat made specific reference to his hospital and approximate date and time of the incident in these posts. The compliance office was concerned that a viewer could reference the post along with easily accessible online news stories and decipher the patient's identity.

Editor: Many programs are only beginning to establish rules around social media with regards to HIPAA, privacy, and security.[1] It might be time to check to see if your policies are up to date before you have a similar incident with one of your learners. Since this is clearly a HIPAA violation, as the patient is potentially identifiable, the learner's behavior falls under the category of poor professional behavior. Programs struggle to clearly identify deficits in the category of professionalism for fear of labelling a learner as unprofessional. Remember, the term "unprofessional" is in reference to their behavior; it is not a permanent judge of their character. In this case the behavior is unequivocally unprofessional.

Pat further infringed upon basic tenets of professional conduct in violating the institution's authorship policy. He authored a case study submission to a national general surgery conference. As a resident physician, the submission form asks for co-authorship from a supervising faculty member. Pat added the residency program director's name to this submission without the director's knowledge or expressed consent.

REMEDIATION APPROACH

All the above-referenced incidents occurred between August and December of Pat's first post-graduate year. As complaints about him came in, the program director met with Pat in an effort to address and mitigate any further problems.

Coaching and counsel on appropriate professional interactions were provided extensively by phone, email, and in-person meetings. The director was hopeful that this one-on-one attention to acknowledge and address the complaints would be enough to improve Pat's behavior.

> *Editor: It is important for the program director to be involved in setting expectations and addressing a struggling learner's academic status and any disciplinary actions. It is unclear if the program director in this case provided the coaching and counseling. Program directors care very much about their residents as people and the success of their residents and their training program. However, they are also in the position, along with a clinical competency committee, of deciding whether or not a resident will graduate. Remediators must engage with their learners on a more personal level; to establish trust and a safe learning environment are absolutely essential. The program director, who makes final decisions about the resident's career success or failure, and who by nature of the position has too many conflicts of interest, must not be the one to conduct remediation.[2,3]*
>
> *While it may not have ultimately changed the outcome, it seems like the program was never able to determine why the learner was behaving this way. This leaves the editor curious as to whether a more in-depth diagnostic evaluation was performed to see if he had other educational challenges. Were his knowledge, clinical reasoning, clinical skills, etc. otherwise up to par? How were his communication and interpersonal skills outside of the clinical setting, such as with his peers in the resident lounge when they were talking about non-work-related topics? Did he have any insight as to whether these were new reactions to his behavior, or had he experienced them in medical school or other settings in his personal life? How far back can he remember being called out for such behaviors? If you can determine the cause of unprofessional behavior, remediation is dramatically more successful.[4]*

However, as Pat's unprofessional behavior escalated to arguing with attending physicians, making social media posts that potentially infringed on patient privacy, and violating the institution's authorship policy, the program leadership recognized the need to begin working with Pat in a more formal and documented manner. In consultation with the institution's clinical competency committee (CCC), program leadership developed a comprehensive remediation plan that included:

1. Attending and successfully completing two classroom instruction courses: "Emotional Intelligence: An Introduction" and "Relationship-Centered Communication," offered by the institution for faculty and professional development.

   Editor: This may work if lack of skill is truly the problem. The editor's prior experience with similar courses is that it really requires a very insightful and motivated learner to implement the content and skills taught in these courses without concurrent coaching of directly observed behavior. It is easy to get through the courses as a passive observer without integrating much of the content into daily practice. These courses lack the active deliberate practice of relevant skills, feedback, and coached reflection that struggling learners require to master new skills.[5]

2. Meeting regularly with an assigned mentor, Dr. Wayne, to discuss techniques to better receive feedback and communicate with colleagues in a professional manner.

   Four critical aspects were worked on throughout their meetings:
   - Professional obligations and expectations during interpersonal communications
   - Understanding the impact of one's behavior on others
   - Clarity of communication and understanding
   - Acceptance of feedback as a way to improve

   Editor: Discussion is helpful, but role playing of techniques on how to better receive feedback and how to communicate with colleagues is critical to change behavior. Consider teaching a learner how to ask for feedback. Rather than asking, "How am I doing?" have the resident identify exactly what they want feedback on, then have them pose a question that does not elicit a judgmental response. For example, don't ask, "How was my interaction with that attending?" Instead, ask, "If you were interacting with that attending, how might you have done it differently?" This will invite more comments from the supervising faculty who can respond without having to judge the learner. The faculty are then more likely to provide valuable feedback, and this adds to the learner's toolbox of performance strategies that can be used in various settings. [4,6]

3. The program leadership actively solicited feedback and written evaluations from attending physicians who, in the course of their regular duties, directly observed conversations between Pat and other providers. Real-time coaching and feedback were given to achieve optimal communication.

    Editor: Real-time coaching and feedback are essential. They must be direct, specific, behavior-based, and the learner must be given a chance for a "do over." [7] If the resident was rude to a physician assistant, they need to apologize and acknowledge that they are in training and trying to learn their role in the culture of medicine. They should ask for permission to try again, at which point they need to repeat the encounter.

4. The program director reviewed and educated Pat on the policies on social media use for both the Accreditation Council of Graduate Medical Education (ACGME) and his institution. Social media outlets were subsequently monitored to ensure no further violations occurred.
5. The research director met with and educated Pat on the institution's authorship policy and reviewed basic professional tenets of scholarly activity.

    Editor: To make these last two requirements more active, Pat could have been asked to research the policies, meet with the director to clarify any concerns, then present what he had learned to his peers. This may also protect against other residents in the program making similar mistakes.

DISCIPLINARY ACTION

Despite attending all classes and meetings and receiving satisfactory evaluations from faculty, Pat's behavior continued to escalate after his remediation plan concluded in the spring of his first post-graduate year. Less than one week after he was removed from remediation, Pat authored another social media post in which he made derogatory comments regarding midlevel providers at his hospital. Readers of the post could clearly identify his name, position, place of work, and department where the incident had occurred. At that time, it was decided by program leadership that his remediation should be reinstated. During this renewed remediation, however, program leadership received formal complaints from patients regarding Pat's behavior. In both incidents, Pat was described as being argumentative and cursing at his patients.

Editor: In this case, remediation was used as a disciplinary action. Based on the editor's experience, many institutions use a warning or probation as disciplinary actions. Some institutions, fearing legal consequences, do not have official policies on remediation or probation.[8,9] This is not recommended.

Remediation is the act of remedying something that is deficient. In and of itself, it does not imply discipline. All people struggle during training in one aspect or another and need additional teaching or coaching. For the majority, their needs are minor; they have insight and are able to seek assistance to correct their deficits without the intervention of program leadership. They do not all warrant disciplinary action. If a learner fails a test because they had the flu while they took the test, which was remediated by studying again and retaking the test, and they go on to pass the test four weeks later, does that warrant disciplinary action? If a learner fails to collect spinal fluid on four consecutive lumbar punctures, then after talking to the chief resident, watching an instructional video on performing the procedure, and seeking out a neurologist to help her perfect her technique, should she be placed on warning? Most would say no.

Think of remediation and disciplinary actions separately. Remediation is supportive, supplemental teaching. Warnings and probation are disciplinary. No program director would be faulted for putting Pat on probation after his second or third incident and in the probation letter stipulating the requirement that he also participate in remediation.

At that time, Pat was immediately placed on an investigatory suspension. Over the ensuing few weeks, the department chair, hospital leadership, and designated institutional officer (DIO) reviewed this resident's case in detail. Additionally, during the investigation, Pat sent an email to the primary investigator providing him with an ultimatum to conclude the inquiry. Compounded by Pat's history of probation for professionalism during medical school, the institution ultimately decided to offer Pat the opportunity to resign in lieu of termination.

SUCCESSES

Though there was some progress and improvement during the initial remediation plan, Pat reverted to prior patterns of problematic behavior once this intensive oversight concluded. He seemed to respond most effectively to the one-on-one meeting with Dr. Wayne. These sessions allowed for a better understanding of Pat's point of view and provided better insight on how to offer advice most effectively. Once it became apparent that Pat's unprofessional behavior and communication deficiencies began to involve patients, formal disciplinary action was taken. The conclusion was drawn that, despite intensive efforts over the course of his first post-graduate year, there was no longer a reasonable expectation that Pat's behavior could be corrected. Ultimately, the resident accepted the offer to resign in lieu of termination.

Editor: When it became apparent that Pat was not able to perform in this program, the program moved swiftly to help him transition to the next phase of his life rather than stringing him along. Sometimes career counseling is provided by remediation faculty. Some exiting learners want to remain in clinical medicine. Some never wanted to be there in the first place, but saddled with debt, can't see that there are other possible career paths. Help learners find a compassionate exit plan.[10] The editor followed up with about 100 learners five years after successful remediation and was surprised to see that a handful had chosen fields outside of clinical medicine, due to career coaching and reflection that had occurred in the trusted conversations between struggling learners and their remediators.[11] Traditionally, underperforming learners continued to practice clinical medicine at higher rates. If Pat continues with his current behaviors, he will never find happiness in medicine. A compassionate remediator can at least help him find some direction in his next life steps.

HINDSIGHT REFLECTIONS FROM THE REMEDIATING FACULTY

Pat demonstrated fundamental deficiencies in professional conduct and interpersonal communication skills. Despite the involvement of multiple parties, his behavior only escalated over the course of his first post-graduate year. One resource we were unable to provide him was any senior residents from whom to model better behavior. As a new program having only enrolled our inaugural class at the time, we were unable to provide any form of mentorship from senior residents. Given that, we may have considered that Pat seek transfer to another program where such a resource was available before disciplinary action needed to be taken. Additionally, red flags were noted as early as Pat's orientation block. The possibility exists that earlier intervention and course-correction following these warning signs could have prevented his behavioral patterns from becoming established – thus providing for a potentially more successful remediation.

Editor: If the learner does seek residency at another location, the editor, who is a strong supporter of struggling learners, asks that you represent his strengths and weakness fairly to any future potential program director. It is in Pat's best interest for future programs to assess whether they have the resources and expertise to assist him with his deficiencies. If you have not read the book Blind Eye: the terrifying story of a doctor who got away with murder *by James B Stewart, please order yourself a copy now.*

REFERENCES

1 Kind T, Genrich G, Sodhi A, Chretien KC. Social media policies at US medical schools. *Med Educ* Online. 2010 Jan 1;15(1):5324.

2 Kalet A, Chou CL, Ellaway RH. To fail is human: remediating remediation in medical education. *Perspect Med Educ.* 2017;6:418-24.

3 Kebaetse MB, Winston K. Physician remediation: accepting and working with complementary conceptualisations. *Med Educ.* 2019;53:210-1.

4 Guerrasio J. *Remediation of the Struggling Medical Learner, 2nd Ed.* Irwin, PA: Association for Hospital Medical Education; 2017.

5   Ericsson KA, Krampe RT, Tesch-Römer C. The role of deliberate practice in the acquisition of expert performance. *Psych Rev.* 1993 Jul;100(3):363.

6   Stone D, Heen S. *Thanks for the Feedback: The science and art of receiving feedback well (even when it is off base, unfair, poorly delivered, and frankly, you're not in the mood).* Penguin; 2015.

7   Hewson MG, Little ML. Giving feedback in medical education: verification of recommended techniques. *JGIM.* 1998 Feb;13(2):111-6

8   Guerrasio J, Furfari KA, Rosenthal LD, Nogar CL, Wray KW, Aagaard EM. Failure to fail: the institutional perspective. *MedTeach.* 2014;36:799-803

9   Weizberg M, Smith JL, Murano T, Silverberg M, Santen SA. What does remediation and probation status mean? A survey of emergency medicine residency program directors. *Acad Emerg Med.* 2015;22:113-6.

10   Chou CL, Kalet A, Costa MJ, et al. Guidelines: The dos, don'ts and don't knows of remediation in medical education. *Perspect Med Educ.* 2019;8:322-338.

11   Guerrasio J, Brooks E, Rumack CM, Christensen A, Aagaard EM. Association of characteristics, deficits, and outcomes of residents placed on probation at one institution, 2002-2012. *Acad Med.* 2016 Mar 1;91(3):382-7.

CASE 5

Professionalism, Communication, Interpersonal Skills, Time Management and Organization, and Clinical Skills

LEARNER AT TIME OF IDENTIFICATION FOR REMEDIATION

Maria, a first post-graduate year psychiatry resident

REASON FOR REMEDIATION

Maria came to the attention of the program leadership for three separate reasons. First, she was recurrently tardy for clinical duties and failed to notify her supervisors. Second, despite clear expectations about completing timely dictations which then needed to be reviewed and finalized, her clinical notes were not completed in the required timeframe after patient encounters. Lastly, Maria struggled with receiving feedback from her rotation supervisors. She displayed unprofessional behaviors and poor interpersonal communication skills such as interrupting during feedback sessions and struggling to ask questions in a respectful manner.

> *Editor: To devise an effective remediation plan, it is exceedingly helpful to know what drives behaviors. For example, a well-meaning faculty member can tell Maria to arrive on time and review the rules, but if they don't know why she is late, they can't help her develop strategies to address the cause of her tardiness. The same applies to her other challenges.*

REMEDIATION APPROACH

The remediation plan, called a corrective action plan, included the following action steps:

1. The program director will communicate directly with Maria's supervisor weekly for the next three blocks regarding:
    a. Punctuality
    b. Dictations performed within 24 hours of examining a patient
    c. Dictations reviewed and finalized within 48 hours of examining a patient
    d. Appropriate acceptance of feedback
2. Improvement benchmarks and timeframe:
    a. The resident will demonstrate improved punctuality and will communicate to her supervising physician and the program administrator at least 10 minutes prior to the start of the clinical day when emergency situations arise
    b. The resident will demonstrate the ability to perform dictations within 24 hours of examining a patient
    c. The resident will demonstrate the ability to review and finalize dictations within 48 hours of examining a patient
    d. The resident will demonstrate openness and acceptance of feedback by not interrupting during feedback sessions and by asking questions at the appropriate time in a respectful manner. The resident will demonstrate the ability to implement the skills she learned from the feedback sessions.
    e. The resident corrective action plan will continue through the rest of her current rotation and her next two rotations

> *Editor: While this plan is filled with what the learner needs to do, there is nothing given to help the learner know **how** to accomplish these skills. Struggling learners typically do not have the ability to self-regulate their learning. They make inappropriate choices on how to improve their performance, often committing more time and effort to trying the same failed strategies, just doing them faster or trying harder – none of which is particularly effective.*[1,2]

If Maria had known how to accomplish these skills, she would have been doing that all along. Nobody wants to fall behind and then feel rushed and get in trouble. She needs strategies that are direct and concrete for how to arrive on time. Where is she coming from – home? Another clinical site? What is causing the delay? This is probably not a new problem, so what has worked for her in the past? Is there a resident who has overcome similar problems that could help mentor her? When should Maria be dictating her notes? Does she spend too much time with patients? Does she need to set a timer to help limit the length of encounters, so she has time to write notes? Does she need a medical and psychiatric evaluation to make sure she doesn't have diseases like attention deficit hyperactivity disorder (ADHD) or narcolepsy that could be causing delays? Does she need to work on her clinical reasoning to help increase her work speed throughout the day? How does one receive feedback? How does one ask for constructive feedback? She needs to be taught new skills to try and be given permission to fail and then try different skills to find what will work best for her.

Maria continued to struggle with accepting feedback in a professional manner. Consequently, she did not successfully remediate her behaviors as outlined in her corrective action plan. She consistently passed her rotations only marginally due to her deficiencies in the areas of professionalism and interpersonal communication skills and was placed on probation.

The probation plan included the following items:

1. The resident will remain on probation for 90 days, during which time the residency program director will communicate with her preceptors on a weekly basis. At the end of three months her status will be re-evaluated.

   Editor: This is standard, but there is no set requirement.

2. The resident's rotations will be modified to a PGY-1 supervision level (at this point she was a PGY-2). She will be removed from any medical

student or resident supervision.

3. The resident will be removed from the Graduate Medical Education Committee.

> *Editor: Removal from extracurricular activities is common.*

4. The program director will contact supervising faculty in the resident's future rotations to encourage a rigorous academic experience emphasizing evaluation and management of common problems (both inpatient and outpatient) as well as issues related to professionalism and interpersonal communication skills.

> *Editor: There is much discussion about the pros and cons of feeding information forward to future supervisors who will also be evaluating the learner. "Feeding forward" of learner information, now being called learner handovers, remains controversial.[3] It is true that learners who are identified as being weaker may suffer from stigmatization, bias, and at times lower expectations.[4] On the other hand, learner handovers also allow for continuity of remedial teaching, continuous and ongoing improvement of skills, the availability of more resources to help the learner, and improved grades.[5,6,7,8,9,10,11] The majority of programs do feed information forward for the betterment of learner education, especially at the residency level where (a) grades have less of an impact on future career progression and (b) ensuring competence as the final step prior to independent practice is more crucial to patient safety. The recommendation is that information be fed forward; that the learner, whether student or resident, is aware of what is being shared and with whom; and that only those who can actively support the remediation efforts be privy to such confidential information.[3]*

5. During each rotation while on probation, the resident will develop a list of 5 commonly managed problems/topics and become facile in discussing each problem/topic with an identified faculty supervisor. The expectation is that she will develop evaluation and management of 15 different problems/topics that represent an evidence-based review of current literature.

Editor: This request is often made of learners with medical knowledge and/or clinical reasoning deficits, rather than time management and organization and inability to accept feedback, which falls under the category problem-based learning and improvement.[12]

6. During the resident's probation period she will be assigned readings from *Professionalism in Psychiatry,* and these chapters will be reviewed with her by various core faculty members to ensure her understanding. The expectation is that the resident will demonstrate understanding of the information by verbalizing her understanding and by implementing the professionalism principles to the satisfaction of the core faculty supervisor and the residency director.

7. During this time, the resident will take calls with backup provided by select core faculty. The resident will learn to demonstrate the ability to safely admit patients into the hospital with the support of core faculty.

8. The resident will be expected to see patients only with direct supervision or indirect supervision immediately available, consistent with PGY-1 supervision. She will actively seek and accept feedback from her faculty supervisor in a professional manner.

9. The resident will be expected to successfully complete a Clinical Skills Verification with a maximum of three attempts on each of the next 3 blocks.

Editor: A Clinical Skills Verification is an exam established by the American Board of Psychiatry and Neurology to be administered by residency training programs. It includes a directed observed assessment of a resident's physician-patient relationship, a psychiatric interview including the mental status exam, and a case presentation.[13]

10. After each block of rotations, the resident will have a one-hour verbal evaluation by 2 faculty members to provide feedback on her performance, plan, and evaluations.

Potential Consequences:

Failure to satisfactorily complete the probation plan or any further evidence of unprofessional behavior may result in dismissal from the residency program or non-renewal of contract.

DISCIPLINARY ACTION

The resident was put on probation after failing to meet all the requirements outlined in the corrective action. She was subsequently able to meet the terms of her probation letter. Presumably due to the detailed steps outlined in the probation plan and the assistance of key personnel, the resident was able to successfully meet the terms outlined in the probation plan, so no further disciplinary action was needed.

SUCCESSES

Strategies that were beneficial in this case included strictly adhering to the timelines for completion and follow-up that were outlined in the corrective action and probation documents, as well as including the program director, associate program director, clinical competency committee chair, supervising faculty, and other key faculty in the process, as all were key personnel in carrying out various steps of the process.

OPPORTUNITIES TO LEARN

A helpful strategy was listening to legal advice to avoid referencing any behavioral health issues in the remediation plans and focusing solely on the deficits related to the resident's job roles. This being a psychiatry program, this advice was valuable as it is generally difficult to exclude behavioral health terminology. The legal advisor did suggest the use of the Employee Assistance Program (EAP), which offered the appropriate resources to support the resident in that way.

> *Editor: All of this is great advice. Program leadership should never put anything in writing that they aren't willing to follow through on. They must avoid using diagnostic language when talking about their learners, even though it is part of our vernacular. Consider all the potential resources when trying to help a learner. Programs have used EAPs, speech and language pathologists, Toastmasters groups, support groups for young adults with high-functioning autism, etc. Think outside the box. What is available through local colleges and in your community?*

HINDSIGHT REFLECTIONS FROM THE REMEDIATING FACULTY

We noticed that the biggest struggles we had during this process directly related to Maria's behavioral deficits. Ultimately, probation was needed to correct those issues. The clinical deficits were more concrete, and remediation was much easier to attain in those areas.

In hindsight, we should have addressed Maria's deficits sooner and put issues in writing earlier on. We received comments from her such as, "Well I've always been doing it this way, and no one said anything before," and "You should have told me sooner." We believe this made it harder to convince her there was a problem and to correct the issues.

Being a new program at the time, we did not have chief residents. However, now that we have chief residents and know how helpful their input can be, had we had them we probably would have solicited their insight and assistance to some degree. 💬

REFERENCES

1   Cleland JA, Arnold R, Chesser A. Failing finals is often a surprise for the student but not the teacher. *Med Teach.* 2005;27:504-8.

2   Patel R, Tarrant C, Bonas S, Yates J, Sandars J. The struggling student: a thematic analysis from the self-regulated learning perspective. *Med Educ.* 2015;49:417-26.

3   Chou CL, Kalet A, Costa MJ, et al. Guidelines: The dos, don'ts and don't knows of remediation in medical education. *Perspect Med Educ.* 2019;8:322-338.

4   Cox SM. "Forward feeding" about students' progress: information on struggling medical students should not be shared among clerkship directors or with students' current teachers. *Acad Med.* 2008;83:801.

5   Gold WL, McArdle P, Federman DD. Should medical school faculty see assessments of students made by previous teachers? *Acad Med.* 2002;77:1096-100.

6   Frellsen SL, Baker EA, Papp KK, Durning SJ. Medical school policies regarding struggling medical students during the internal medicine clerkships: results of a national survey. *Acad Med*. 2008;83:876-81.

7   Price JA. Sharing student background information with faculty: does it make a difference? Dissertation, Harvard University;2012.

8   Cleary L. "Forward feeding" about students' progress: the case for longitudinal, progressive, and shared assessment of medical students. *Acad Med*. 2008;83:800.

9   Cohen GS, Blumberg P. Investigating whether teachers should be given assessments of students made by previous teachers. *Acad Med*. 1991;66:288-9.

10   Pangaro L. "Forward feeding" about students' progress: more information will enable better policy. *Acad Med*. 2008;83:802-3.

11   Warm EJ, Englander R, Pereira A, Barach P. Improving learner handovers in medical education. *Acad Med*. 2017;92:927-31.

12   Carraccio C, Wolfsthal SD, Englander R, Ferentz K, Martin C. Shifting paradigms: from Flexner to competencies. *Acad Med*. 2002 May 1;77(5):361-7.

13   Dalack GW, Jibson MD. Clinical skills verification, formative feedback, and psychiatry residency trainees. *Acad Psych*. 2012 Mar 1;36(2):122-5.

CASE 6

Clinical Reasoning and Communication

LEARNER AT TIME OF IDENTIFICATION FOR REMEDIATION

Anton, second year out of medical school as a second-year house medical officer (international case)

> *Editor: Being a house officer is a general year of training comprised of rotations in general medicine, surgery, emergency medicine, and other general medical specialties.*

REASON FOR REMEDIATION

Anton came to the attention of program leadership because his medical team noticed that he had difficulty in presenting clinical cases to consultants, too often getting bogged down in details. The senior medical staff would then get frustrated, as it was difficult for them to understand what the most salient points were so they could develop their own opinion about each case. It was equally difficult ascertaining what Anton believed to be the medical problem with the patients and how he thought the patients should be diagnosed and treated.

REMEDIATION APPROACH

Anton's remediation lasted a total of 4 months and was conducted by the director of clinical training (DCT). The DCT is the medical specialist (similar to an attending physician) working with the medical education unit (similar to a resident and fellow team and teaching staff).

1. The DCT met with Anton to discuss his role and how he could assist Anton with his performance and development. The DCT started by genuinely inquiring about Anton's perspective on the problem and explored underlying reasons. Anton believed he just got "overwhelmed" with presentations and was perplexed that the level of detail he provided was not getting him positive recognition. He knew "something wasn't right," but couldn't articulate what it was.

   Editor: Early learners commonly hold this misconception. They don't understand why more doesn't equate to better. They think more information will demonstrate that they are hardworking and dedicated, and they feel that they should be rewarded. Sometimes this can be fixed by simply recalibrating expectations that the learners should collect and present the most relevant information rather than the greatest volume of information.

2. The DCT then worked to determine the root cause of the presentation issues.

   • First, the DCT tried to clarify whether or not there was a problem with Anton's knowledge, his assessment (history/examination) skills, clinical reasoning, or presentation skills. By working through some examples of common clinical cases, he was able to prove that Anton had good medical knowledge and could derive differentials well, but he collected (and tried to present) an overwhelming volume of information.

   • Second, the DCT determined what/if any schemas were being used for clinical reasoning or presentation. He asked Anton to try using a structured SOAP approach (subjective, objective, assessment, then plan). Anton found this simple to use and showed he could derive a useful list of differential diagnoses. However, the volume of information he gave was huge and all-encompassing (at times irrelevant), and he struggled to commit to a likely diagnosis or initial management plan. With more practice, Anton found the SOAP format simple and effective in improving how to identify key information to present.

- The DCT then worked with him on advanced application of schemas in simulated clinical case discussions for different audiences. They reviewed the needs of various audiences and how to tailor key information accordingly.

Editor: This is such a valuable thing to teach. Many of our struggling learners, regardless of the domain in which they are deficient, demonstrate a lack of flexibility.[1] Every case gets the same presentation, regardless of the complexity, specialty, and urgency. The style of every communication interaction is the same whether they are talking to a peer in the lounge, their supervisor, or a patient. Struggling learners need to be taught what is culturally expected in different situations. In this case, what an emergency department doctor needs to hear about a patient is very different from a neurologist, which is very different from a family medicine doctor.

- Next, the DCT took on various roles such as the ED physician, orthopedic surgeon, or rehabilitation physician. This identified that Anton had difficulty discriminating what was needed for different presentations, and so would give all the information, irrespective of the relevance or intended audience

Editor: Active practice is crucial to learning and encoding new skills.[2]

3. Simulation

- The DCT then coached Anton on identifying the most relevant information for each unit. By doing this, Anton was able to adapt his SOAP presentation.
- This was the focus for many sessions.

Editor: Working with struggling learners takes patience because it takes a lot of time. There are many scenarios to review, and some learners need to review scenarios repeatedly before the lesson becomes ingrained.[3,4,5,6]

4. Contextualizing learning – real cases

- Once Anton was doing well with simulated simple cases, he progressed to replicating real cases he had seen in clinical practice. He would present them to the DCT, who would role play a variety of different relevant roles. This learning strategy was key in building Anton's competence and confidence, incorporating reflection into his practice.

Editor: These sessions seem rich with opportunities for feedback, for reflection, and for practicing new skills in a safe environment – the 3 key steps of deliberate practice![2] *Any chance to build a learner's self-efficacy contributes to motivation, willingness to participate, and both short- and long-term academic performance improvements.*[7,8]

DISCIPLINARY ACTION

None

SUCCESSES

From Anton's perspective: "Having been asked what my personal goals were, and then having an interaction based off that, was critical. I feel as if working in a flexible time with the education unit was super, and I sometimes came in on my days off. …Having just the right amount of attention was ideal: not too many eyes glaring into my soul, just the few that would help me get better at being a doctor."

When asked sometime later if he benefited from remediation, Anton said, "I do now feel like a safer doctor. I'm appreciative that you guys were there for me at my lowest. I absolutely love my job and wouldn't feel the same way if it wasn't for you guys demonstrating that someone cares."

Editor: Getting learner feedback is a great idea. It will help teaching faculty and institutions improve their remediation process and skills, and the responses may truly surprise everyone. Learners once thought to have no insight will return to thank you with profound realizations. Learners who seemed disgruntled throughout the entire process will, surprisingly, be genuinely grateful.[9]

HINDSIGHT REFLECTIONS FROM THE REMEDIATING FACULTY

We wondered if remediation stopped a bit too early as he showed such great improvement. We know that he would have benefitted from more time. At this juncture we also wonder how long the improvement will be sustained.

We think one of the most valuable aspects shown in this case is the importance of developing a trusting coaching relationship so that the learner can be vulnerable and at the same time feel safe.

Editor: Ideally everyone would be offered the one-on-one learner-centered teaching that remediation provides, but clearly the resources are not available for this level of intense education. Likewise, remediation can only last so long. At some point, learners need a chance to test out the new skills they have learned to see if they will be successful as independent providers. Programs too often fail to reassess learners after remediation to ensure that it was successful.[10] *Progress, motivation, and some insight are a great place to launch once post-remediation assessments have validated improvement of skills to a level of at least minimal competence for the learners' level of training.*

REFERENCES

1   Kalet A, Chou CL. *Remediation in Medical Education.* New York: Springer; 2014.

2   Ericsson KA, Krampe RT, Tesch-Römer C. The role of deliberate practice in the acquisition of expert performance. *Psych Rev.* 1993 Jul;100(3):363.

3   Guerrasio J, Garrity MJ, Aagaard EM. Learner deficits and academic outcomes of medical students, residents, fellows, and attending physicians referred to a remediation program, 2006-2012. *Acad Med.* 2014 Feb 1;89(2):352-8.

4   Guerrasio J, Aagaard EM. Methods and outcomes for the remediation of clinical reasoning. *JGME*. 2014 Dec 1;29(12):1607-14.

5   Warburton KM, Goren E, Dine CJ. Comprehensive assessment of struggling learners referred to a graduate medical education remediation program. *JGME*. 2017 Dec;9(6):763-7.

6   Zbieranowski I, Takahashi SG, Verma S, Spadafora SM. Remediation of residents in difficulty: a retrospective 10-year review of the experience of a postgraduate board of examiners. *Acad Med*. 2013 Jan 1;88(1):111-6.

7   Stegers Jager KM, Cohen Schotanus J, Themmen AP. Motivation, learning strategies, participation and medical school performance. *Med Educ*. 2012;46:678-88.

8   Malau-Aduli BS, Page W, Cooling N, Turner R. Impact of self-efficacy beliefs on short- and long-term academic improvements for underperforming medical students. *Am J Educ Research*. 2013;1(6):168-176.

9   Guerrasio J, Aagaard EM. Long-term outcomes of a simulation-based remediation for residents and faculty with unprofessional behavior. *JGME*. 2018 Dec;10(6):693-7.

10   Hawthorne MR, Chretien KC, Torre D, Chheda SG. Redemonstration without remediation – a missed opportunity? A national survey of internal medicine clerkship directors. *Med Educ Online*. 2014;19:25991.

CASE 7

Mental Well-Being

LEARNER AT TIME OF IDENTIFICATION FOR REMEDIATION

Mandy, first year out of medical school as a first-year house medical officer (international case)

> *Editor: Internship is a general year comprised of 3 core rotations (general medicine, surgery, and emergency medicine) and 2 other rotations (mental health, radiology, or others).*

REASON FOR REMEDIATION

Mandy came to the attention of program leadership because of her frequent absences from work and anxiety, both of which compromised her performance and led to extended time completing tasks and staying late every day.

REMEDIATION APPROACH

Mandy's remediation was conducted by the director of clinical training (DCT). The DCT is the medical specialist (similar to attending physician) working with the medical education unit (similar to a resident and fellow team and teaching staff).

1. The DCT met with Mandy to discuss his role and to talk to Mandy about her challenges. Mandy did not identify that she struggled with

anxious feelings, or that her performance was being impacted by her well-being. However, the DCT found that she often had a shaky voice and got "stuck" on small details which made it at times difficult for conversations to progress. The DCT thought their discussions had "resolved" some of the supervising physician's concerns, but Mandy continued to dwell on what she thought she "should have done better."

2. When the DCT had conversations about the benefits of seeking professional help, Mandy showed reluctance. However, when she heard the recommendation was for her to work with an elite sports psychologist who typically worked with talented sportspeople needing to perform under a great deal of pressure, akin to junior doctors, Mandy was more receptive.

> *Editor: It is disheartening to realize and acknowledge that stigma still exists around psychiatric care and mental health treatment in the medical community. This is especially true given how many trainees and practicing clinicians who are not in need of remedial teaching seek mental health services for their own well-being.[1] While many struggling learners feel like they are the only ones in need of mental health support, in the editor's experience, the vast majority will seek help at some point during training and again while in independent practice. Hours are spent trying to de-stigmatize care seeking and pave the way for struggling learners to access mental health care. The idea of approaching mental health from the perspective of sports psychology is a very creative invitation to treatment and may increase the learner's level of engagement as well.[2] One study demonstrated that students who had pursued sports previously and had presumably been exposed to sports psychology had less burnout, less maladaptive behaviors, and improved well-being as medical students.[3] Some also use the analogy of a life coach or executive business coach, many of whom are trained in psychology.*

3. The education department funded an initial set number of consultations, and they worked with the psychologist to come up with an agreed-upon plan.

- The advice from the psychologist was for the DCT to continue offering support and guidance to help performance under pressure, rather than finding solutions to reduce psychological discomfort (e.g. taking a break, reducing load). Whilst reducing load/taking a break might be a viable option to help Mandy, it was advised that it should not be seen as an immediate mechanism to solve a problem. The primary goal was in capacity building, not symptom reduction.
- The psychologist would focus on capacity building as opposed to symptom reduction, so that the priority for Mandy and the education team was on functioning and performance quality (that is, fulfilling the job role). The goal was not for Mandy never to feel anxious or pressured, but rather to create a work environment that promoted increased capacity to tolerate and embrace those uncomfortable emotions.
- The DCT and her psychologist checked in by catching up with, listening to, and empathizing with Mandy. This was critical to building her capacity as struggles were to be normalized and treated compassionately.

DISCIPLINARY ACTION

None

SUCCESSES

Mandy was extremely pleased with the sports psychologist's intervention and admitted that she would not have participated had it not been funded by the education unit. She was surprised how effective and useful it was and reported significant improvement to her performance and well-being. Having realized the value, Mandy said she would continue to self-fund the intervention after the initial visits. The key things that helped Mandy were: (a) recognizing the impact anxiety was having on her performance, (b) shifting away from blaming herself for what she perceived as errors to using strategies such as reframing situations and challenges, and (c) incorporating breathing techniques throughout a workday.

Editor: This is another great example of understanding the perspective of the learner, thinking outside the box, and utilizing all the resources available in one's community. Just getting her started on a path in which she noticed an improvement will keep her motivated and engaged. This is common with struggling learners. We are often looking for big gains, whereas they notice the small gains and use them to propel themselves forward and to trust in our guidance and recommendations. ᠗

REFERENCES

1   Wallace JE. Mental health and stigma in the medical profession. *Health.* 2012 Jan;16(1):3-18.

2   Cocks M, Moulton CA, Luu S, Cil T. What surgeons can learn from athletes: mental practice in sports and surgery. *Journal of Surgical Education.* 2014 Mar 1;71(2):262-9.

3   Babenko O, Mosewich A. In sport and now in medical school: examining students' well-being and motivations for learning. *Intl J Med Educ.* 2017;8:336.

CASE 8

Professionalism, Time Management and Organization, Medical Knowledge, Clinical Skills, Clinical Reasoning, and Mental Well-Being

LEARNER AT TIME OF IDENTIFICATION FOR REMEDIATION

Alana, first year out of medical school as a first-year house medical officer (international case)

> *Editor: Internship is a general year comprised of 3 core rotations (general medicine, surgery, and emergency medicine) and 2 other rotations (mental health, radiology, or others).*

REASON FOR REMEDIATION

Due to her low academic scores at the university where she did her medical school training, Alana was already on the radar before she was referred for remediation. Because of this red flag, direct observation of clinical skills occurred prior to the commencement of her internship. This enabled a learning plan to be developed and shared with the junior doctor and the relevant education unit supervisors during the pre-employment period. Based on that information, considerations were made such as thoughtful placement of her within a more supportive unit team to facilitate transition from medical student to medical practitioner. She was also encouraged to use her long commute times to listen to podcasts to improve her medical knowledge. Her initial progress was slow.

Editor: Some residents do arrive with known "red flags" such as poor exam scores, low grades on clinical rotations, and prior probationary status.[1,2] Some students come from colleges, medical schools, or prior training programs that are either known to be weak or are completely unknown. The editor learned from communicating with hundreds of programs that those which routinely take higher-risk residents often put their new residents through a simulated or live exam (observed structured clinical encounter or mini-clinical examination) to assess their incoming skills and derive an individualized learning plan for each learner from the start of their training.

The editor also learned while visiting programs around the world that a few program directors interview all their learners after they have been accepted into their training programs and ask, "Do you anticipate having any learning or performance challenges while in training?" Most learners who will go on to struggle are able to identify their areas of weakness in this initial encounter, but not necessarily the severity of the weakness. This has allowed some programs to shore up support early on or help learners access the necessary resources sooner rather than later.

While on her first rotation, emergency medicine, Alana saw and evaluated patients who presented emergently to a metropolitan hospital. While being directly observed providing clinical assessment of her patients, her evaluators identified (1) a suboptimal knowledge base, (2) substandard procedural skills, and (3) disorganized clinical assessment skills. Specifically, Alana lacked a structured approach to history gathering, and she had a disorganized, non-systematic physical examination process.

Once referred for remedial teaching, the director of clinical training (DCT) also identified other challenges. Alana could not synthesize cases, had poor clinical reasoning, and therefore couldn't present cases. In addition, her energy, time, and mental capacity for medicine and her education were distracted by trying to maintain a personal business while being a trainee, undergoing IVF treatments, and spending 2-3 hours commuting to and from the clinical sites each day.

Editor: While this learner seems to be struggling with all possible performance deficits, it is important to determine which deficits are driving all her struggles.[3] However, if you say to her that she is failing in all domains and needs to fix everything, that will crush her spirit and she will likely feel as if she is facing an insurmountable obstacle. Can the problems be narrowed down? For one, if she doesn't have knowledge, there is no way she can synthesize cases and therefore her ability to clinically reason through cases has yet to be truly tested. Is the disorganization driving her inability to learn and present? Are the distractions outside of her education too demanding and outcompeting the needs of her career? Maybe all the factors are present, but is there a main contributor on which to place focus for remediation?[4]

Alana then received an "unsatisfactory" overall midterm assessment on her first rotation from the unit supervisor.

REMEDIATION APPROACH

Alana's remediation was conducted by the DCT, who was allocated to provide Alana with support and co-ordination of her education. The DCT is the medical specialist (attending physician) working with the medical education unit (resident team and teaching staff). This remediation lasted the duration of the first year.

Fortunately, after the first "unsatisfactory" mark, Alana had the insight that she needed to reconsider her life's priorities. This translated to high prioritization of her medical career over other commitments and renewed effort and commitment to the remediation process. The DCT noticed greater engagement from the junior doctor and more motivation to improve.

1. First, there was direct observation by the DCT of Alana's clinical skills to determine her individual learning needs and to develop a learning plan(s) to address those needs.
2. The DCT then prioritized all available supports, taking into consideration the multiple clinical deficits and external factors that impact clinical work.
3. Metropolitan rotations were chosen over rural rotations to allow ongoing supervision by the DCT.

4. Education units worked to optimize orientation and expectations at each new site. It was made clear that Alana was expected to attend all orientations.

5. Early and regular contact by the DCT with the rotation site leader assisted with optimizing local support (e.g., considering any local/ unit hurdles such as composition of team members, allocation of one education unit supervisor for the duration of rotation, having more senior trainees directly supervising the intern, early and regular unit registrar feedback, etc.).

6. Alana was encouraged to be proactive in seeking feedback to address concerns early, all with the purpose of facilitating her growth.

7. Tailored support strategies were given by way of explicit learning plan(s) (developed by the DCT) for each rotation with involvement of all stakeholders (i.e Alana, rotation site director, and education supervisor).

8. Regular contact with Alana was maintained to monitor implementation or challenges implementing the learning plan. Having regular DCT catch-ups with Alana helped with monitoring progress, allowed reflection from all parties to be reviewed with Alana, and permitted further tailoring and finessing of her learning plan going forward.

9. The educational unit gave regular feedback on Alana's progress.

10. Frequent testing of medical knowledge (by online quizzes) was given to assess baseline and to highlight areas for personal study.

11. Regular case-based discussions were held to develop an organized and structured clinical approach. Clinical reasoning and identification of when to escalate concerns were promoted.

12. The learning plans were regularly updated to remain dynamic and tailored to Alana's individual progress/needs.

13. Regular reflection by the junior doctor was encouraged.

By mid-year, this intern had shown she could maintain a consistent "satisfactory" level of performance. Following this, a period of autonomy was fostered by gradually having the intern "lead" and "plan" aspects of the remediation process, such as number of DCT catch-ups, types of cases to present, and topics for discussion. In the final rotation of the year, DCT supervision was only used when required.

DISCIPLINARY ACTION

None

> *Editor: There are no guidelines as to when a learner should be placed on a letter of academic warning or probation. Given the amount of time and faculty resources that were put into this learner, most programs would have placed her on some form of disciplinary action – if not probation, at least a letter of warning or the equivalent. Many programs only use probation if the problem is related to the academic competency of professionalism, which may be short-sighted. Consider this: if you think that there is a chance that the learner will not complete the year on time, or that the learner will not graduate from your program, then placing that learner on a letter of warning or probation is both legally prudent and fair to the learner. While a learner doesn't want to know that they may get kicked out of a program, it is already on their mind, and they will generally appreciate transparent communication about the process. Many residents think that they could lose their job at any minute for any minor mistake and need reassurance if that is not the case. The other reason to place a learner on probation is if you think they need to be identified after they graduate as someone who may need to be watched for recurrence of their struggles.*

SUCCESSES

Some of the most successful strategies were to intervene early on with the education units of each rotation to "optimize" the local working environment and to document learning plans with explicit objectives, key learning goals, and key milestones with dates to serve as reminders.

Regular DCT contact with both the education units and Alana helped reenforce and actualize early high-quality feedback. Regular quizzes highlighted Alana's areas for improvement.

OPPORTUNITIES TO LEARN

In the beginning, the DCT reminded Alana too often of what needed to be done. This may have delayed her personal development as an independent professional.

HINDSIGHT REFLECTIONS FROM THE REMEDIATING FACULTY

We should have allocated more responsibility of learning to the junior doctor earlier.

Editor: Never give more than 110% of the effort that the struggling learner is giving. In this case, she seemed to have insight and was willing to adapt her life and practices…but it is still a good lesson. Don't try so hard to make your remediation efforts or program successful that you start doing the work for the learner or provide so much structure that without you they fall apart again. Finding that balance is the art of remediation.

REFERENCES

1   Harfmann KL, Zirwas MJ. Can performance in medical school predict performance in residency? A compilation and review of correlative studies. *J Am Acad Derm.* 2011 Nov 1;65(5):1010-22.

2   Papadakis MA, Arnold GK, Blank LL, Holmboe ES, Lipner RS. Performance during internal medicine residency training and subsequent disciplinary action by state licensing boards. *Ann In Med.* 2008 Jun 3;148(11):869-76.

3   Guerrasio J, Garrity MJ, Aagaard EM. Learner deficits and academic outcomes of medical students, residents, fellows, and attending physicians referred to a remediation program, 2006-2012. *Acad Med.* 2014 Feb 1;89(2):352-8.

4   Guerrasio J. *Remediation of the Struggling Medical Learner, 2nd Ed.* Irwin, PA: Association for Hospital Medical Education; 2017.

CASE 9

Communication, Interpersonal Skills, Professionalism, and Practice-Based Learning and Improvement

LEARNER AT TIME OF IDENTIFICATION FOR REMEDIATION

Brian, assistant professor of pediatrics

REASON FOR REMEDIATION

Complaints were received by the residency's program evaluation committee (PEC) for persistent negative teaching evaluations and potential faculty verbal mistreatment/abuse of residents. The faculty member reportedly berated residents for prolonged periods of time for what many residents perceived as minor details – e.g., not keeping up on the details of the handoff list for patients, not having a complete list of patient medications, etc.

> *Editor: For those who have provided remedial teaching to students, residents, fellows, and faculty, it quickly becomes apparent that the techniques for remediation are the same.[1,2] Motivations and the process may vary a bit, but the overall structure of remediation – from identification, to diagnosis, to devising a remediation plan – are the same. The approach to a faculty member who speaks inappropriately to residents who are perceived as being incompetent is no different from the resident who speaks inappropriately to nurses who are perceived as being incompetent.*

REMEDIATION APPROACH

Despite Brian having received feedback from the residency's program director (PD) and departmental chair, concerns about his interpersonal and communication skills persisted. He was removed from the teaching service by the PD on the recommendation of the residency's program evaluation committee (PEC). The PEC also advised that Brian be appointed to a faculty coach. He was referred to a senior faculty member in another department who had experience with remediating struggling learners, including faculty.

The faculty coach approached the situation using a 4-step framework by Iobst and Holmboe[3]: (1) problem identification, (2) problem investigation and classification, (3) determination of an appropriate intervention, and (4) assessment of the success (or not) of the intervention.

Problem Identification: Initially, the main challenge reported was within the competency of interpersonal and communication skills, which at times was also interpreted to reflect unprofessional role modeling for a teaching faculty (e.g., berating a resident for prolonged periods of time for not having complete details of a patient's medication list).

Problem Investigation and Classification: Prior to meeting with Brian, the faculty coach sought feedback from the PD and departmental chair about specific incidents of lapses in interpersonal skills and communication. To maintain confidentiality, the coach did not speak directly to residents or other faculty in the department because Brian had been a faculty member in the department for several years prior. The faculty coach also inquired about other possible non-work-related issues that might be impacting Brian's workplace and his environment using the "7 Ds" of non-work-related impairments.[3] (See **Table 9.1**) None were apparent, and Brian remained otherwise highly productive both clinically and academically, without any other reported interpersonal or communication incidents with patients or other health-related professionals with whom he worked.

Editor: People who provide remedial teaching often refer to themselves as coaches. And while that term may be more palatable, the role is fundamentally different, with some overlapping features. A coach typically partners with a client with the goal of posing thought-provoking questions that inspire a creative process to maximize the client's personal and professional potential. The coach honors the client as the expert and helps them set their own goals. With remedial teaching, the remediator is often working with a learner that lacks insight, doesn't see the feedback surrounding them, and doesn't know how to implement feedback or set new practice goals for themselves. The remediator is the expert in teaching and learning. He or she takes a much more active role in helping the learner to identify deficits, seek and see feedback, and learn how to change practice so as to implement feedback. Like a coach, the remediator also gives emotional support and encouragement and guides the process. Rarely is a true coach successful in remediating a learner.

The faculty coach then met with Brian to hear his side of the current situation, carefully maintaining an open mind before making any decisions and realizing that intentions and behaviors are not often congruent.[4] The faculty coach also inquired directly about the "7 Ds", but these alternative factors seemed unlikely. Brian affirmed his enjoyment of teaching, his disappointment at the current situation, and his earnest desire to return to the teaching service. He emphasized that his intention in rebuking residents for not keeping up the patient handoff lists or not having patients' complete medication lists was to instill good habits in young trainees and optimize quality patient care. Brian appeared somewhat taken aback to hear about the poor evaluations since he actively sought feedback, and the feedback he recalled receiving from residents was mostly positive. The faculty coach concluded that the competencies involved included not only interpersonal and communication skills resulting in reported unprofessional behaviors (e.g., berating residents), but also practice-based learning and improvement (e.g., partial resistance in accepting feedback).

Editor: Struggling learners universally have trouble receiving feedback, and there are several reasons for this. First, it is very difficult to give critical corrective feedback, so those giving the feedback tend to be vague, less direct, and sometimes bury it too deeply in other content for it to raise to any level of awareness. Second, knowing that Brian will be evaluating them makes it harder for residents to give feedback up the chain of hierarchy.

Feedback, however, is not only verbal, and it exists everywhere. Even without verbal feedback, most people (not in need of remediation) sense when they need to adjust their behavior and do so consciously or unconsciously based on non-verbal cues.[5] On the receiver end, struggling learners do not pick up on non-verbal feedback. They don't learn from the hidden curriculum. They can't decipher abstract feedback. They don't see feedback that is embedded in other content. And even when they receive feedback, they don't know how to actualize the information or change their practice to improve their performance. The person providing feedback MUST point out that their message is intended to be feedback; provide it verbally in clear, direct, succinct language; and offer a corresponding alternative action plan. "When you encounter this specific situation (describe), instead of doing X, try doing Y."[2,6]

Like giving feedback, learning how to accept feedback is also an art. Encourage learners to listen to feedback and try to understand it without defending their actions. Think of feedback as adding tools to your skills toolbox. How can this tool or strategy that I have been given be used again in my future practice? For faculty who are requesting feedback from their students, the editor suggests asking the learner to think about the best attending that they ever had and then ask, "What were some of the things that that attending did that you really liked?" This is much easier for a student to respond to than asking them to describe how their supervisor personally could be better. Remind learners that feedback is a gift from someone who cares enough to want to help you improve upon your practice. It is much easier to tell you that you are doing fine and to walk away.[2,6] Don't forget to thank the giver of feedback. It can be a hard job.

The faculty coach decided that a coaching approach emphasizing appreciative inquiry best fit the situation.[7] To build trust in the relationship, the coach informed Brian that he (the coach) would not participate in any summative decisions about his case with the PD and departmental chair and that all conversations would remain confidential.[8] Since Brian appeared well-intentioned and motivated to change, the faculty coach decided to first approach the issue by focusing on enhancing Brian's insight and reflective capacity for the current situation.[9,10] He informed Brian this process could take time – months, possibly years – which Brian readily acknowledged and guaranteed his willingness and commitment to change and improve. Emphasis on deliberate practice, feedback, and informed self-assessment formed the three key pillars of this remediation program.[2]

Editor: Trust is so important, and the separation of the coach from any decisions regarding teaching privileges is crucial.

Determining an Appropriate Intervention: To facilitate insight and reflective capacity, the faculty coach asked Brian insightful questions such as, "What will you do if you are not permitted back on the resident teaching service?" Brian's initial response was that teaching was so important to him as a physician that he might consider moving to other teaching institutions in the area. The faculty coach then inquired, "If you move to another teaching institution, do you think these same concerns might arise there as well? And if not, why not?" Followed by, "What makes the current situation different from other teaching institutions?" Brian was then asked to complete a 9-item reflective professional identity essay.[11] (See **Table 9.2**) Subsequent discussions were utilized to facilitate and impress upon him the seriousness of his current situation. At the same time, using appreciative inquiry, the dialogue also facilitated potential solutions that aligned with the faculty's goal to return Brian to the faculty teaching service.

Editor: In this instance, the learner and institution had the same motivating goals: both wanted Brian to be able to teach. Note that only behaviors and performance need to be aligned, not necessarily the motivating goals of the struggling learner and the remediation faculty or the institution. When motivations are not aligned, the challenge is to find what truly motivates the learner and to use that to engage them in changing their behaviors.

In bi-weekly meetings, lengthy discussions on feedback and the challenges of self-assessment were held. Five articles were assigned to Brian to read, reflect, write about, and discuss with the faculty coach.[12,13,14,15,16] In addition to appreciative inquiry, the faculty coach used the frameworks of growth mindset[17] and self-determination theory to guide the in-person discussions.[18,19,20] (See **Table 9.3**) Self-determination theory is a broad underlying theory of human motivation based on fulfilling the 3 basic psychological needs of autonomy, competency (or mastery), and relatedness (or a sense of purpose). To facilitate autonomy, the faculty coach asked Brian how *might* (rather than *should*) these 5 articles apply to himself.[20] Brian's sense of competency was encouraged by emphasizing that being a good teacher takes deliberate practice and building of reflective capacity.[21] Relatedness was supported by aligning these sessions with Brian's strong desire to be a part of an academic teaching institution. Throughout the conversations, emphasis was placed on changing the misdirected behaviors and purposefully avoiding personalizing the feedback to the individual self.[17,19] For example, instead of saying, "You are a bad teacher for yelling at your residents who forget to update the patient handoff list," the faculty coach would emphasize, "Yelling is a behavior that can be changed to better reflect your intention of high-quality patient care." These discussions helped Brian gain further insight into the limitations of self-assessment in isolation and the credibility of the residency feedback being offered.

> *Editor: Growth mindset exists on a continuum with fixed mindset and can be thought of in the context of resiliency and the ability to persevere through educational challenges. People with a fixed mindset see mistakes, challenges, and setback as signs of stupidity and incompetence and are quicker to give up.[22] People with a growth mindset see mistakes, challenges, and setbacks as opportunities to learn and become better clinicians. This is admittedly a bit simplistic and more for demonstration purposes, but if you agree with the notion that "everyone is a certain kind of person and that there's not much they can really do to change that," you're more of a fixed-mindset sort of person. If you are more likely to agree that "people can substantially change the kind of person they are," you tend toward the growth-mindset type.*

After a few weeks, the faculty coach and Brian felt good progress was occurring. However, another incident occurred of a similar nature which was a surprise to Brian. The faculty coach reaffirmed that changing unintentional habits may be difficult and take time. But he also felt there had to be a change in Brian's reflective capacity – moving from reflection *on* action (i.e., reflecting after the fact on intentional or unintentional behaviors) to reflection *in* action (i.e., increasing situational awareness and reflective insight of unintentional behaviors that may be occurring in the moment).[10] To promote this greater awareness, Brian was asked to read the book *Emotional Intelligence 2.0* and take the online self-assessment instrument.[23] The faculty coach met with Brian to discuss how this topic might apply to him. Brian realized he "wears his emotions on his sleeve" and that at times such emotions may become misperceived by others. He also realized that weekend calls were often very busy and stressful, and these days became high-risk periods of unintentionally unprofessional behavior with learners. In *Emotional Intelligence 2.0*, 4 core emotional intelligence skills are delineated: self-awareness, self-management, social awareness, and relationship management. Within each skill, specific strategies are identified. (See **Table 9.4**) Each week Brian was asked to choose one strategy to work on and report back to the faculty coach how successful (or not) he was in accomplishing this goal.

To promote reflection *in* action, Brian was asked to email his faculty coach as soon as possible with any potential incident of behavior that he thought might be misperceived by resident learners. It was emphasized that waiting to hear reports from the program evaluation committee of further interpersonal communication incidents was too late, since the event had already occurred. The following is an example of such an email exchange:

Brian's initial email: Earlier today I was in a conversation with another attending physician during clinic. The other attending was having a tough day and was venting to me. A second-year resident came up to present a patient. Given the sensitivity of the discussion, I told Anthony, the resident, to give us a few minutes to continue this conversation in private, and he left. I thought this was handled with courtesy in a polite tone but is it possible that this request may have been misinterpreted.

Faculty mentor's email response: I appreciate your rapid attention to increase your situational awareness. I think the key is HOW you said it to the resident – tone, inflection, etc. Remember what the research says, we don't really "hear" ourselves speaking. We think we do but the superior temporal sulcus – that part of our brains that interprets language – shuts down when we are speaking so we don't really "hear" how we really sound. Perhaps one approach to take is to follow up with Anthony and simply explain to him that you were having a private conversation with another attending physician and see if he understands. Explain it was not intended to be dismissive or curt to him. See how the resident reacts and what he says.

Brian email the next day: I spoke with Anthony today in follow-up. He said he had no problem with the message nor how it was said. He completely understood and felt the tone/inflection were all fine and added that he wanted me to know that "I have never felt you treated me inappropriately ever." It sounded very genuine, but we've talked about the difficulty in getting honest feedback given the hierarchy of medicine.

I had a text interaction today with another resident, Timothy. He updated me on a patient to let me know he was going to follow up with the social worker who was working on the discharge disposition. My initial text reply was the social worker already called me yesterday. I immediately thought that Timothy might think this could be a dig that the social worker called me already because he might not be doing his job. I promptly sent a second text clarifying to let him know the social worker reached out to me without calling any residents because she wanted to verify the discharge date plan directly from me and not because a resident wasn't returning her page. I'm trying to turn that superior temporal sulcus on!

Faculty Mentor's response: Great job – that superior temporal sulcus is getting a workout! I like how you were proactive, thought about how the situation might be misperceived, and then sent a second page to clarify the situation with Timothy.

Assessment of the Intervention: About 8 months after the initial meeting, the faculty mentor and Brian mutually agreed to halt the in-person monthly meetings but remain in contact via email for any future incidents or opportunities for discussion. About a year later, the faculty coach reached out to see how things were going. Brian felt the situation was much improved, citing specific incidents of positive feedback from resident learners and the residency program director.

DISCIPLINARY ACTION

Removal of the faculty member from the departmental teaching services by the program director upon the recommendation from the PEC.

> *Editor: One of the most difficult decisions to make is when to return a faculty member such as Brian to a teaching service. While each learner is different, the more experience one has working with struggling learners, the better they become at making the decisions that rely more on the art of remediation rather than the evidence-based science. There will never be a set time frame as to*

when someone is ready to resume their duties. Patient safety is usually the marker as to when someone can resume practice or resume certain activities with more autonomy. In Brian's case, the safety of the learning environment is at stake. Does the struggling faculty member need to successfully pass observed structured teaching encounters (OSTEs)? Do they need to demonstrate satisfactory skills while being directly observed with students and residents? Is it up to the coach to determine whether the struggling faculty is ready to return or to have their skills reassessed? The former is not recommended, while the latter is preferred. Too often programs fail to reassess struggling learners and ensure that remediation was successful prior to allowing them to resume roles.[24,25]

SUCCESSES

Nearly 3 years later, Brian continues to do well, and no further incidents have been reported to the residency's program evaluation committee. He remains a committed teacher, is fully integrated into the teaching program of the department and has been promoted to associate professor in the clinician educator track. This track recognizes faculty for their clinical care, scholarly activities, and reputation as a teacher with excellent learner evaluations. 💬

TABLE 9.1   The Seven Ds of Non-work Related Impairment[3]

1. **Distracted** (e.g. family and relationships, financial, etc.)

2. **Depression**

3. **Drugs** and substance abuse

4. Learning **Disorders** (e.g. attention deficit-hyperactivity disorders, autism spectrum disorders, slow reading rate, etc.)

5. **Deprivation** of sleep

6. **Disease** (acute or chronic medical illnesses)

7. Personality **Disorders**

TABLE 9.2 Professional Identity Essay[11]

---

1. What does being a member of the medical profession mean to you? How did you come to this understanding?

2. What do you expect of yourself as you work towards becoming a full-fledged physician?

3. What will patients expect of you?

4. What will the profession expect of you? How did you come to this understanding?

5. What conflicts do you experience or expect to experience between your responsibility to yourself and others, e.g., patients, family, profession? How do you resolve them?

6. What would be the worst aspect for you if you failed to live up to the expectations you have set for yourself?

7. What would be the worst aspect for you if you failed to live up the expectations of your patients?

8. What would be the worst aspect for you if you failed to live up to what society expects of physicians? How did you come to this understanding?

9. Think of a physician you consider to be an exemplar of professionalism. Describe why you chose this person, illustrating with an incident or pattern of decisions or actions that support your choice.

TABLE 9.3 Coaching Tips that Promote Self-Determination Theory's Three Basic Psychological Needs of Human Motivation[18-20]

Basic Psychological Need	Approaches that Foster / Promote
Autonomy	• Take other's perspective (e.g. ask the learner for his/her views of what they want to learn) • Provide choices • Provide a meaningful rationale when choices cannot be offered • Minimize controlling words » Avoid "ought," "need to," "must," and "should" since they decrease sense of autonomy » Instead, use phrases like "you *can* learn this, maybe you *could* do it this way, it *would* help to include this in your study." » Instead of, "I will tell you what you need to do next," ask, "How do you think you should handle it next time?"
Competency (Mastery)	• Set an optimal level of challenge (i.e., "just-right" degree of difficulty; know your audience) • Support the skills development necessary to meet the posed challenge (by providing the right combination of experiences, conditions, and tools to master the task at hand) • Give meaningful feedback framed positively toward the achievement of competence » Negative feedback can undermine a sense of competence and cause demotivation » Positive feedback that is merely praise can be harmful » Give positive feedback that helps the individual recognize gains in competency and performance and identifies the next step to further mastery » Shift the focus of the feedback from the individual to the context/task (e.g., instead of, "You failed to do this," say, "This case/skill/procedure is difficult. Let's see how to get there.")
Relatedness (Sense of Purpose)	• Acknowledge feelings and convey empathy • Create structure to foster individual connections (e.g., by facilitating the formation of interpersonal relationships with representatives of the institutional culture) • Create structures to foster group and community connections (e.g., foster students' sense of themselves as a cohesive group or class)

TABLE 9.4   **Core Skills and Suggested Strategies as Adapted from** *Emotional Intelligence 2.0* [23]

(Please see the book *Emotional Intelligence 2.0* for a more comprehensive list)

What I See	What I Do
Self-Awareness Strategies:	
1. Quit considering feelings as either good or bad	**Self-Management Strategies:**
2. Observe the consequences of your emotions	1. Correct your breathing
3. Sit with and understand your discomfort	2. Exchange reasons for emotions
4. Feel your emotions with your body	3. Announce your goals
5. Know who and what are your emotional triggers	4. Count to ten
6. Observe yourself	5. Sleep on decisions and thoughts
7. Journal about your emotions	6. Talk to a skilled coach
8. Understand your bad moods	7. Smile and laugh and do it again
9. Understand your good moods, too	8. Create time for problem solving
10. Consider why you behave the way you do	9. Manage your self-talk
	10. Imagine yourself achieving your goals

PERSONAL COMPETENCE

What I See	What I Do
Social Awareness Strategies:	**Relationship Management Strategies:**
1. Address people by name	1. Be open and be curious as to why
2. Pay attention to body language	2. Don't change your style; enhance it
3. Understand that timing is everything	3. Are you giving mixed signals?
4. Have something prepared to discuss	4. Model accepting feedback
5. Consider whether you should take notes at meetings	5. Be reliable and trustworthy
6. Plan ahead for events	6. Be available
7. De-clutter your life	7. Only get angry intentionally
8. Live in the moment	8. Don't avoid conflict
9. Pay attention to emotional quotient (EQ) at the movies	9. Acknowledge emotions in others
10. Practice being a good listener	10. Show your care, if it is genuine

SOCIAL COMPETENCE

REFERENCES

1   Guerrasio J, Aagaard EM. Methods and outcomes for the remediation of clinical reasoning. *JGIM*. 2014 Dec 1;29(12):1607-14.

2   Guerrasio J. *Remediation of the Struggling Medical Learner, 2nd Ed.* Irwin, PA: Association for Hospital Medical Education; 2017.

3   Iobst W, Holmboe ES: Chapter 15. The learner with a problem or the problem learner? Working with dyscompetent learners. In: Holmboe ES, Durning SJ, Hawkins RE (editors) *Practical Guide to the Evaluation of Clinical Competence*. Philadelphia, PA. Elsevier. 2nd Edition. 2018. Pages 288-302.

4   Rees CE, Knight LV. The trouble with assessing students' professionalism: theoretical insights from sociocognitive psychology. *Acad Med*. 2007 Jan;82(1):46-50.

5   Hewson MG, Little ML. Giving feedback in medical education: verification of recommended techniques. *JGIM*. 1998 Feb;13(2):111-6.

6   Stone D, Heen S. *Thanks for the Feedback: The science and art of receiving feedback well (even when it is off base, unfair, poorly delivered, and frankly, you're not in the mood)*. Penguin; 2015.

7   Deiorio NM, Carney PA, Kahl LE, Bonura EM, Juve AM. Coaching: a new model for academic and career achievement. *Med Educ Online*. 2016 Dec 1;21:33480.

8   Chou CL, Kalet A, Costa MJ, Cleland J, Winston K. Guidelines: The dos, don'ts and don't knows of remediation in medical education. *Perspect Med Educ*. 2019 Dec;8(6):322-338.

9   Hays RB, Jolly BC, Caldon LJ, McCrorie P, McAvoy PA, McManus IC, Rethans JJ. Is insight important? Measuring capacity to change performance. *Med Educ*. 2002 Oct;36(10):965-71.

10   Schon DA: *The Reflective Practitioner: How professionals think in action*. New York, NY. Basic Books. 1983.

11   Bebeau MJ, Faber-Langendoen K: Remediating lapses in professionalism. In: Kalet A, Chou CL (editors) *Remediation in Medical Education. A mid-course correction*. New York. Springer 2014. Pages 103-127.

12   Bing-You RG, Trowbridge RL. Why medical educators may be failing at feedback. *JAMA*. 2009 Sep 23;302(12):1330-1

13   Sargeant J, Mann K, van der Vleuten C, Metsemakers J. "Directed" self-assessment: practice and feedback within a social context. *J Contin Educ Health Prof*. 2008 Winter;28(1):47-54.

14   Davis DA, Mazmanian PE, Fordis M, Van Harrison R, Thorpe KE, Perrier L. Accuracy of physician self-assessment compared with observed measures of competence: a systematic review. *JAMA*. 2006 Sep 6;296(9):1094-102.

15   Kruger J, Dunning D. Unskilled and unaware of it: how difficulties in recognizing one's own incompetence lead to inflated self-assessments. *J Pers Soc Psychol*. 1999 Dec;77(6):1121-34.

16   Mizrahi T. Managing medical mistakes: ideology, insularity and accountability among internists-in-training. *Soc Sci Med*. 1984;19(2):135-46.

17   Ramani S, Könings KD, Ginsburg S, van der Vleuten CPM. Twelve tips to promote a feedback culture with a growth mind-set: Swinging the feedback pendulum from recipes to relationships. *Med Teach*. 2019 Jun;41(6):625-631.

18   Lyness JM, Lurie SJ, Ward DS, Mooney CJ, Lambert DR. Engaging students and faculty: implications of self-determination theory for teachers and leaders in academic medicine. *BMC Med Educ.* 2013 Nov 11;13:151.

19   Ryan RM, Deci EL: Self-determination theory and the facilitation of intrinsic motivation, social development and well-being. *Amer Psychol.* 2000;55:68-78.

20   Kusurkar RA, Croiset G, Ten Cate TJ. Twelve tips to stimulate intrinsic motivation in students through autonomy-supportive classroom teaching derived from self-determination theory. *Med Teach.* 2011;33(12):978-82.

21   Srinivasan M, Li ST, Meyers FJ, Pratt DD, Collins JB, Braddock C, Skeff KM, West DC, Henderson M, Hales RE, Hilty DM. "Teaching as a Competency": competencies for medical educators. *Acad Med.* 2011 Oct;86(10):1211-20.

22   Dweck C. What having a "growth mindset" actually means. *Harvard Business Review.* 2016 Jan 13;13:213-26.

23   Bradberry T, Greaves J: *Emotional intelligence 2.0.* San Diego, CA. TalentSmart®. 2009.

24   Hawthorne MR, Chretien KC, Torre D, Chheda SG. Redemonstration without remediation – a missed opportunity? A national survey of internal medicine clerkship directors. *Med Educ Online.* 2014;19:25991.

25   Chou CL, Kalet A, Costa MJ, et al. Guidelines: The dos, don'ts and don't knows of remediation in medical education. *Perspect Med Educ.* 2019;8:322-338.

CASE 10

Professionalism and Interpersonal Skills

LEARNER AT TIME OF IDENTIFICATION FOR REMEDIATION

Jasmin, a second-year physician assistant student

REASON FOR REMEDIATION

Jasmin was a second-year physician assistant (PA) student when she failed her pediatrics rotation. She stated that during the rotation she thought she was doing "okay," but acknowledged that there were a few interactions with nurses and nurse practitioners that went poorly. She did not realize she was at risk of failing or even underperforming until she received a failing grade at the end of her rotation. Comments about Jasmin on the preceptor evaluation included:

- "frequent interruption of others during sign out"
- "mocked me, the attending physician"
- "had no respect for the flow of the day and did not act as if she was visitor or student, but rather an attending who had been there for 20 years and should just have everyone's respect"
- "very judgmental about some of the parents' social situations"
- "seemed uninterested in taking patients she felt were not complex enough for her time or effort"

Editor: Many professional schools that start with didactic curriculum for the first half hear rumors about students who "will likely have problems on their clinical rotations" or who are already struggling with professionalism and interpersonal skills. The curriculum, however, is often designed to test only knowledge. Opportunities to assess and evaluate professionalism and interpersonal skills are missed. Small-group activities provide ample occasions for faculty and peers to assess and provide feedback and for faculty to formally evaluate these skills. Unless professionalism, communication, and interpersonal skills are evaluated in a way similar to skills like medical knowledge, students will view them as less important or merely perfunctory. Was there an opportunity earlier in Jasmin's training, prior to her receiving an "F" on a clinical rotation, to identify these challenges, set expectations, and begin remediation? It is costly and difficult to repeat rotations, and failing grades on transcripts can dramatically affect students' career opportunities. Failing grades are necessary to communicate competence, and certainly not everyone deserves to pass, but remediation prior to evaluation is ideal to give the learner a better chance to succeed.

A study some years ago looked at the accuracy of the rumor mill in identifying struggling learners; it was found to be 98% accurate.[1] Consider this. If remediation were not thought of as a punishment, but instead merely as mentorship and additional teaching, then by reacting to the rumor mill we would be able to identify struggling learners much earlier. In the worst-case scenario, 2% of identified learners would receive additional one-on-one teaching that they didn't necessarily need but would still benefit from.

REMEDIATION APPROACH

The remediation team created for Jasmine consisted of two PA school faculty members and one faculty member with more expertise in remediation. The team met with Jasmin and developed remediation objectives and an implementation plan. At bi-weekly meetings, they discussed the objectives and reflected on what was going well and what could use improvement. The time course of the remediation was 4 months.

Remediation Objectives:

1. Discuss how professionalism facilitates or hinders patient care
2. Identify triggers that may cause you to behave in ways that others may perceive as unprofessional
3. Discuss how you will become aware when you are triggered
4. Discuss how you will manage triggers that change your behavior
5. Identify potential sources of professionalism feedback
6. Discuss how lapses of professionalism could negatively affect your career as a PA
7. Discuss how successful remediation of lapses in professionalism may impact your career as a PA
8. Interview one person with a different socioeconomic background from yours
9. Discuss the barriers to care, social determinants of health, and health disparities faced by a patient that you met during your rural rotation
10. Develop a plan with your remediation team on how to approach others for feedback
11. Incorporate feedback you receive on professionalism into your daily practice
12. Demonstrate professional behavior during the remediation process

Editor: These objectives capture all 3 components of deliberate practice – practice, feedback, and reflection – and allow for depth in their development.[2] For example, 2 and 3 are great reflection objectives, and 4 allows the learner to identify and adapt her behaviors. 5, 10 and 11 home in on receiving feedback. The editor conducted a study that showed a simulation remediation that focused on principles of deliberate practice very similar to these was 90% effective in correcting unprofessional behaviors in residents and faculty for at least 2-4 years.

Remediation Implementation Plan:

1. Meet with the remediation team
2. Complete an essay describing objectives 2-9
3. Utilize 3 journal articles for objectives 6 and 7

4. Have professionalism evaluations filled out by the supervising provider and ancillary staff every 2 weeks while on rotations
5. Review professionalism evaluations with a member of the remediation team
6. Participate in a videotaped standardized or simulated case to assess professionalism
7. Spend 8 hours volunteering at the local free medical clinic
8. Consider utilizing outside resources such as student services or campus mental health resources for support

DISCIPLINARY ACTION

Due to her poor professional behavior, Jasmin was placed on academic probation and required to repeat the pediatrics clinical rotation. She was allowed to continue her previously scheduled rotations while participating in an individualized structured remediation plan and registering for a 1-credit-hour independent study course. Because she had to repeat the pediatrics rotation, her graduation was delayed.

Editor: Probation is the unofficial standard disciplinary action when a learner fails a course. It is also recommended when graduation is delayed.

It is at the school's discretion whether to let the student continue to the next rotation once they have a failure on their transcript. Consider stopping a learner to conduct remediation before the learner accrues more failing grades and additional rotations that will need to be repeated. If you think that the learner will likely be successful while completing the additional demands of the remediation plan, then it is fair to let them proceed. For example, if a student failed the internal medicine exam, but is going on to family medicine next, he or she may be able to remediate the exam as the content is similar. However, if the student failed an internal medicine exam and is moving on to neurology, don't set them up to fail neurology because they are trying to study for a make-up internal medicine exam while trying to study for their neurology rotation at the same time.

SUCCESSES

Using the plan outlined above, Jasmin was able to identify that she was more prone to exhibiting unprofessional behavior during times of stress. She identified that these situations were often due to an unfulfilled need such as sleep, validation, acceptance, or due to anxiety. Using self-reflection, she identified ways to help prevent unprofessional behavior and adopted the motto "management starts with prevention." Jasmin was also able to identify that she was anxious and needed help to manage her anxiety. She began doing daily meditation coupled with weekly therapy. She met with her preceptors weekly to discuss her performance including professionalism and reviewed the feedback with her remediation team. Jasmin completed the remediation plan outlined above. There were no further lapses in professionalism during the remainder of her time in school. The remediation team felt that she was successfully remediated in the deficit of professionalism and ultimately went on to graduate without further incident.

HINDSIGHT REFLECTIONS FROM THE REMEDIATING FACULTY

We are not sure that it was a good idea to ask the student to research journal articles regarding remediation. We think that self-reflection would have been sufficient. If we had felt it was necessary to talk to the student about the studies, we should have brought the articles to her to discuss in a remediation meeting.

> *Editor: This is a valuable reflection. Our learners' time is limited, and how we want them to spend that time requires much consideration. As leaders in remediation we are always learning for our future learners.* ⌨

REFERENCES

1   Rosenthal MM. *The Incompetent Doctor: Behind closed doors.* McGraw Hill. 1995.

2   Ericsson KA, Krampe RT, Tesch-Römer C. The role of deliberate practice in the acquisition of expert performance. *Psych Rev.* 1993 Jul;100(3):363.

CASE 11

Professionalism

LEARNER AT TIME OF IDENTIFICATION FOR REMEDIATION

Dawn, a second-year physician assistant student

REASON FOR REMEDIATION

While on a family medicine rotation, Dawn frequently cared for and became close with Alex, a 6-year-old patient who had autism, and his family. Without permission from Alex's parents, Dawn posted a picture of herself and Alex on Facebook with a caption describing the patient's medical condition. The patient's father saw the picture and caption on Facebook, contacted Dawn (who immediately took the photo off Facebook), and contacted her program.

> *Editor: Like the case of Pat earlier (Case 4), Dawn behaved unprofessionally with regards to her use of social media. Unprofessional behavior has been described as students displaying content of self-intoxication, illegal drug use, posting of patient information, and racist content.[1] No two cases are alike. This appears to be Dawn's only infraction, while Pat had a long list and ended up resigning. Let's see if this case has a different end result.*

REMEDIATION APPROACH

A remediation team was created for Dawn consisting of a team of 2 PA school faculty members and one faculty member with more expertise in remediation. The remediation team met with her and developed remediation objectives and an implementation plan. They all met bi-weekly to discuss the objectives and reflect on what was going well and what could use improvement. The remediation lasted two months.

Remediation objectives:

1. Discuss the legal and regulatory requirements of PA students and PAs with regard to patient confidentiality
2. Describe your own lapse in professionalism
3. Identify stakeholders who are impacted by lapses in professionalism
4. Describe how lapses in professionalism impact relationships with stakeholders
5. Describe how technology can influence the principles of ethical practice, informed consent, and professional growth
6. Demonstrate professional behavior during remediation

Implementation plan:

1. Meet with the remediation team regularly (bi-weekly)
2. Complete an essay describing Objectives 1-5
3. Submit to a professionalism evaluation from preceptors during the remediation time period and review evaluations with remediation team
4. Meet with a HIPAA compliance officer to assist you in preparing a teaching session on HIPAA compliance
5. Deliver teaching session to peers regarding HIPAA compliance

Editor: All medical professionals make mistakes from time to time, and we all rely on our peers for education – most often in the form of medical consultation. Having a learner teach their peers ensures that the struggling learner has read the rules and regulations regarding social media use and understands them well enough to teach them to others. This will hopefully prevent peers from making the same mistake, and the struggling learner may be humbled by indirectly or directly acknowledging their errors publicly.

Some programs require learners to write letters of apology to all those involved and submit them to the remediation team or their mentor. In this case, Dawn wrote a letter to the patient's family and the dean for negatively representing and influencing the reputation of the program. These letters are not to be critiqued, but are to be used to gauge the learner's professional development. Nor are they actually sent to the involved parties, as the wording may not seem genuine or be legally appropriate. One learner reported that, at first, having to write the letters changed his behavior so he wouldn't have to keep writing letters; eventually he came to understand through writing the letters the greater impact of his behavior. Again, these letters were never corrected, and he never received direct feedback on their content. It was his own "journaling" and developmental process that led to his insight. No one can force their perspective or values onto another.

In her book Learning from Lapses, *Dr. Mak-van der Vossen recommends that 10 questions be asked of learners who behave unprofessionally:* [2]

1. *What happened?*
2. *Do you agree with the unprofessional behavior judgement?*
3. *What did you intend to do?*
4. *What did you expect to happen?*
5. *What circumstances influenced your behavior?*
6. *Were you able to influence the circumstances?*
7. *What do you think your behavior did to others?*
8. *How do you feel about it now?*
9. *Are there any circumstances that make it more difficult for you than for others to comply with professionalism expectations?*
10. *How would you act in a similar situation next time?*

DISCIPLINARY ACTION

Dawn was placed on academic probation during her remediation process.

SUCCESSES

The self-reflection and essay writing worked extremely well for this student. Dawn gained significant insight into her breach of confidentiality and understanding of HIPAA. She also gained excellent feedback from fellow students on her HIPAA compliance teaching session.

HINDSIGHT REFLECTIONS FROM THE REMEDIATING FACULTY

We don't think there is much we would have done differently.

Editor: Sometimes our students are very well intentioned but make mistakes because of their youth and immaturity. Dawn is the type of student who likely took her mistake very seriously, felt terrible about it once she understood the broader ramifications (or will over time), and will never make this mistake again. This stands in sharp contrast to Pat from Case 4, who had multiple professionalism violations of escalating concern.

Dr. Mak-van der Vossen classifies unprofessional behavior into 3 categories: (1) accidental – the learner behaves unprofessionally by accident and is capable of preventing future professionalism lapses, (2) gaming or struggling – the learner experiences difficulty acting professionally, (3) disavowing – the learner refuses to acknowledge repeated unprofessional behavior despite remedial teaching. For the accidental learner, Dr. Mak-van der Vossen recommends exploring the behavior with the learner, understanding their behavior, and teaching them. For the gaming or struggling learner, she recommends remediation and that the learner be followed attentively. For the disavowing learner, she suggests gathering evidence for dismissal and strictly monitoring the learner until their dismissal. 💬

REFERENCES

1   Barlow CJ, Morrison S, Stephens HO, Jenkins E, Bailey MJ, Pilcher D. Unprofessional behaviour on social media by medical students. *Medical Journal of Australia*. 2015 Dec;203(11):439.

2   Mak-van der Vossen M. *Learning from Lapses: How to identify, classify and respond to unprofessional behaviour in medical students*. Amsterdam: Gildeprint; 2019.

CASE 12

Clinical Reasoning

LEARNER AT TIME OF IDENTIFICATION FOR REMEDIATION

Jack, end of the year first-year resident in internal medicine

REASON FOR REMEDIATION

Jack was referred to the centralized coaching and remediation program by his program director (PD) in light of concerns expressed by supervising faculty and peer evaluations. On a recent intensive care unit (ICU) rotation, it was noted that Jack often failed to respond appropriately to urgent situations. He required a lot of supervision during the management of acutely ill patients, and his evaluators noted that he struggled to identify "sick versus not sick." It was noted that he "lacks ownership of patients, particularly in critical situations," "struggles to prioritize clinical information," and is "overwhelmed by complex patients." His medical knowledge, as assessed by prior standardized test scores, and his command of factual information observed on rounds in the intensive care unit the previous month, is slightly above average. He has good organizational systems for completing his daily work. He is enjoying residency and denies any concerns related to mental well-being. There were no other concerns related to professionalism.

> *Editor: The ICU is a common location for identifying clinical reasoning deficits.[1] Patients who present to the hospital are often given a preliminary diagnosis with a list of differential diagnoses in the emergency department.*

By contrast, outpatient-based care frequently involves management of chronic illnesses or new problems with ample time to look up differential diagnoses. In the ICU, a patient's status changes rapidly and requires interns to be able to quickly make their own differential diagnoses and work up patients without the support of others. In addition, the supervising resident is often less available, off tending to other patients or doing procedures.

It is also important to point out that the institution that submitted this case has a remediation program that is centralized on the campus. Most centralized programs (and there are only a few) work with struggling medical students, residents, and fellows across all disciplines and faculty. They are able to gain expertise via their increased exposure to struggling learners and have consolidated access to resources and a team for support.[2,3] Data has shown that remediation success correlates to the experience of the faculty conducting the remediation.[4,5] Whenever possible, a centralized model should be considered.

REMEDIATION APPROACH

The institution's clinical reasoning coaching program involves three phases:

Phase 1 – Learners are referred to the centralized coaching and remediation program, either by their program director or by self-referral. A remediation specialist performs a standardized assessment, using a biopsychosocial approach, that consists of reviewing available evaluative data and performance in prior programs, followed by a face-to-face interview with the learner. A primary clinical performance deficit is identified, chosen from the following categories: medical knowledge, clinical reasoning, organization/efficiency, professionalism, communication, or operative skill. For those with a primary clinical reasoning deficit, the learner moves to Phase 2.

Phase 2 – Learners with a primary clinical reasoning deficit are referred to a clinical reasoning coach to initiate a clinical reasoning remediation program.

The author of this case, whom we will call Dr. Ginsburg, worked with Jack as his primary clinical reasoning coach. They met 11 times (60 minutes each) over a period of 5 months, one-on-one, in person, in Dr. Ginsburg's office. The coaching sessions, which Dr. Ginsburg spent 18 hours preparing for, opened with a discussion of learner expectations and goals including a self-assessment of Jack's strengths and weaknesses. Then they reviewed key clinical reasoning concepts and terminology. Between coaching sessions, Jack reviewed articles, online videos, and cases to solidify these concepts. The following is a list of the resources provided:

Review Articles:

1. White coats and fingerprints: diagnostic reasoning in medicine and investigative methods of fictional detectives.
   https://www.ncbi.nlm.nih.gov/pmc/articles/PMC1322237/
2. Slowing down when you should: a new model of expert judgment.
   https://www.ncbi.nlm.nih.gov/pubmed/17895673
3. Cognitive load theory in health professional education: design principles and strategies.
   https://www.ncbi.nlm.nih.gov/pubmed/20078759

Videos:

- Organizing Knowledge and Information.
  https://www.youtube.com/watch?v=Xo6tXmTYwdA
- Forward Thinking and Pattern Recognition Require Better Problem Representation.
  https://www.youtube.com/watch?v=BMjABNHTw-g
- Forward Thinking: Narrowing the Differential Diagnosis Possibilities.
  https://www.youtube.com/watch?v=ctbGlSNngw0
- Illness Scripts. https://www.youtube.com/watch?v=KATky6USI6E
- How to Create an Accurate Differential Diagnosis from a Patient's Presentation: An Intern Level Case.
  https://www.youtube.com/watch?v=n48zY7GLqc0

Cases:

1. Problem representation: A 43-Year-Old Woman with Abdominal Pain and Fever.
   https://www.ncbi.nlm.nih.gov/pmc/articles/PMC2896582/

2. Illness scripts: A 22-Year-Old Woman with Abdominal Pain. https://www.ncbi.nlm.nih.gov/pmc/articles/PMC4061356/
3. Generating and prioritizing a differential diagnosis: NSTEMI or Not: A 59-Year-Old Man with Chest Pain and Troponin Elevation. https://www.ncbi.nlm.nih.gov/pmc/articles/PMC3599030/

The first session began with an introduction to the clinical reasoning pathway (**Figure 12.1**), a linear stepwise progression of diagnostic and management reasoning processes: hypothesis generation, data collection, problem representation, refinement of hypotheses, development of a working diagnosis (script selection), and management. Though the simplicity and linear nature of this pathway is not completely realistic, this process allows the coach to identify specific deficits amenable to targeted intervention. Jack was asked to methodically work through cases in this stepwise fashion, with repeated prompting from the coach to think aloud.

FIGURE 12.1

Linear clinical reasoning pathway used for targeted remediation

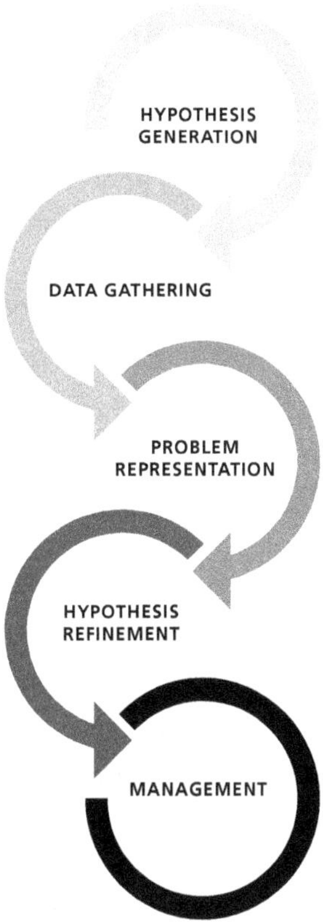

HYPOTHESIS GENERATION

DATA GATHERING

PROBLEM REPRESENTATION

HYPOTHESIS REFINEMENT

MANAGEMENT

This process allowed the coach to identify specific deficits amenable to targeted intervention. Then, during semi-weekly one-on-one, case-based sessions, a systematic approach was provided for each step along the pathway. For example, Jack was encouraged to use System-2-based schema in generating an early, broad differential diagnosis.

> *Editor: System 1 refers to implicit, automatic, pattern recognition decision making, or nonanalytical reasoning. System 2 refers to explicit, controlled, rational, effortful, relatively slow analytical reasoning.*[6]

Pre-test Probability
Consider the probability of suspected diseases, based on their prevalence, specific to a given patient. Common diseases are common.

Anatomical
What lives there? Consider the organs and surrounding structures in a given location and what can go wrong with each.

Pathophysiology
Consider the physiological processes of disease leading to the chief complaint.

Systems
Consider various organ systems and disease processes in each.

Worst-Case Scenario
Consider conditions that can lead to mortality or significant morbidity specific to a given patient. These are "can-not-miss" diagnoses.

Jack lacked a structured approach to any and all clinical presentations of disease. He relied on his relatively strong base of medical knowledge and, unknowingly, overly relied on System 1 thinking. To combat this, he and Dr. Ginsburg worked systematically and analytically through numerous cases, varying the clinical focus for each. The goals of these case-based exercises were to promote metacognition and to instill a systematic, structured, hypothesis-driven process with which Jack could approach a given case. Jack took a thoughtful and respectful approach to these coaching sessions. He showed up on time to each session and put forth strong effort. He completed all assigned tasks.

In most cases, Jack was able to identify key features of a history and physical (H&P) specific to the working differential. When cases were clinically straightforward, he was able to modify and reprioritize his data gathering as new information was revealed. He actively compared and contrasted diagnostic considerations based on case features. After repeated practice with this schema, he developed appropriately broad differentials including the worst-case scenario and assigned appropriate weighting to items on the differential. His oral presentations were usually easy to follow and well organized. As cognitive load increased due to case complexity and/or urgency, Jack struggled to maintain focus and at times became overwhelmed with new, conflicting case data. In these instances, presentations became somewhat circumferential. With more complex clinical scenarios, he was not consistently presenting a brief, highly synthesized clinical case, extending beyond the available features to a search for missing elements.

To improve this, focus was placed on hypothesis-driven data collection. A script search exercise was practiced during each case. For each specific chief complaint, Jack was asked to generate a broad differential diagnosis, then prompted to gather only five history items and three physical exam findings. This exercise forced the learner to consider differentiating and distinguishing features of each diagnosis. Dr. Ginsburg then asked Jack to compare and contrast key features of each diagnosis. This exercise was repeated for multiple chief complaints. Finally, Dr. Ginsburg provided Jack with fully written H&Ps for unfamiliar patients and asked him to highlight key features of the histories and physical exams while reading the notes from beginning to end. Again, this exercise focused on identification of differentiating and distinguishing features of a case while simultaneously considering multiple diagnoses.

Jack's difficulty combating cognitive load also likely explained his poor performance during urgent patient scenarios. To combat this, they practiced using a management script template. Providing a management script template, an educational scaffold of potential types of interventions, can augment the first challenging step of identifying what a clinician might do. The use of a management script template forces the learner to consider all the potential management options for a given diagnosis. (See **Table 12.1**) Then, Dr. Ginsburg asked Jack to select which interventions to perform (i.e., management option selection) based on patient-specific characteristics. This encapsulates the inherent uncertainty and nuance of management decision-making and requires consideration of high-value care, testing and treatment thresholds, prognosis, and risk. Furthermore, urgent clinical encounters typically require management decisions prior to creation of a refined differential diagnosis. In these cases, the patient's clinical response to management interventions, specifically testing and treatment, may guide prioritization of the differential diagnosis. Although Dr. Ginsburg's coaching focused extensively on System 2-derived analytical approaches to hypothesis generation, these can be of limited use in urgent clinical encounters because they are inherently slow. Use of the management script template allowed Jack to create a broad list of potential management options from which to select interventions. Dr. Ginsburg discussed with Jack the benefits and risks of each management option specific to a given patient using fictional, though realistic, urgent situations he would likely experience on the internal medicine wards (e.g., shortness of breath, tachypnea, hypoxia; hypotension and tachycardia). In addition to management planning and diagnostic reasoning, these coaching sessions asked Jack to work slowly, step-by-step through his thought process and communication with each member of the healthcare team in a given scenario.

Finally, Dr. Ginsburg asked Jack to keep a log of all the calls he received from nurses during a shift or call cycle. Dr. Ginsburg then asked Jack to reflect on the calls after the shift and assign a level of urgency from 1-6. This allowed Dr. Ginsburg to review specific incidents in which Jack failed to recognize urgency and explore the reasoning that led to this failure in more detail. With repeated practice, Jack's ability to discriminate "sick" from "not-sick" improved. He was able to describe the steps he would take in common urgent situations and improved at assessing his own level of uncertainty.

Phase 3 – Lessons learned through work with the clinical reasoning coach were then fed forward to faculty and/or peer evaluators for use during subsequent direct observation in the clinical learning environment. Building on data from the global and targeted assessment of the learner, the coach gathered real-time feedback from these evaluators and, when necessary, provided education regarding the assessment and coaching of clinical reasoning in the clinical learning environment.

TABLE 12.1 Example Management Script Template Worksheet

	All Management Options for Diagnosis/Syndrome	Patient-specific management selection
LABORATORY STUDIES		
IMAGING STUDIES		
PROCEDURES		
CONSULTS		
MEDICATIONS		
MONITORING		

This program has developed an interdepartmental clinical reasoning coaching committee in an effort to train members in a standardized approach to the diagnosis and coaching of clinical reasoning deficits among graduate medical learners and to develop durable materials that a variety of academic departments at the institution can use for coaching. In Jack's case, the clinical reasoning coach worked with future supervising faculty evaluators to transition the coaching program to the department level in Phase 3.

DISCIPLINARY ACTION

None. Referral to this program is a pre-disciplinary process.

SUCCESSES

The program was successful. Jack went on to do relatively well in residency and was ultimately hired as a hospitalist at a community hospital.

HINDSIGHT REFLECTIONS FROM THE REMEDIATING FACULTY

In hindsight, we wish we had had an evidence-based assessment and coaching tool to help learners like Jack who struggle with urgent situations. Our clinical reasoning coaching program, and we assume most others, relies on one-on-one meetings in a calm environment conducive to a slower, more methodical and reflective approach to diagnostic and management decisions. In our experience, this approach is usually ineffective for coaching clinical reasoning in urgent situations where, by definition, stress levels are higher and the importance of each decision is magnified. Coaching this learner spurred a greater focus on this phenotype of clinical reasoning struggle within our remediation program.

Editor: The editor has had a very similar experience and success remediating clinical reasoning. Among all the deficits observed in struggling learners, clinical reasoning along with communication deficits take the most time to remediate because numerous one-on-one meetings are required to go over a wide variety of cases.[2] Simply reading cases doesn't impart the complexity of the clinical reasoning process to learners struggling with this deficit. This remediation team discussed and reviewed more complex concepts with its learners than the editor has reviewed with learners during remediation of clinical reasoning in the past.[7] Simplification of more complex terminology and concepts, based on their experience as represented in this case, does not appear to be necessary.

Lastly, while the editor was successful in remediating learners with this deficit to competent, she was never able to bring a struggling learner from well below average to above average. Most learners settle out around the mean or just below after the completion of remediation. It is unclear if the subtle differences in this technique as compared to those described in JGIM*'s "Methods and outcomes for the remediation of clinical reasoning"[7] would help a learner reach a higher benchmark of competence.* 📖

REFERENCES

1   Kalet A, Chou CL. *Remediation in Medical Education.* New York: Springer; 2014.

2   Guerrasio J, Garrity MJ, Aagaard EM. Learner deficits and academic outcomes of medical students, residents, fellows, and attending physicians referred to a remediation program, 2006-2012. *Acad Med.* 2014 Feb 1;89(2):352-8.

3   Guerrasio J. *Remediation of the Struggling Medical Learner, 2nd Ed.* Irwin, PA: Association for Hospital Medical Education; 2017.

4   Winston KA, van der Vleuten CP, Scherpbier AJ. The role of the teacher in remediating at risk medical students. *Med Teach.* 2013;34:e732-42.

5   Winston KA, van der Vleuten CP, Scherpbier AJ. Prediction and prevention of failure: An early intervention to assist at-risk medical students. *Med Teach.* 2014 Jan 1;36(1):25-31.

6   Kahneman D. A perspective on judgment and choice: mapping bounded rationality. *Am Psychol.* 2003; 58(9):697-720.

7   Guerrasio J, Aagaard EM. Methods and outcomes for the remediation of clinical reasoning. *JGIM.* 2014 Dec 1;29(12):1607-14.

CASE 13

Clinical Reasoning

LEARNER AT TIME OF IDENTIFICATION FOR REMEDIATION

Alvarez, a fourth-year medical student

REASON FOR REMEDIATION

Alvarez was referred to his institution's centralized coaching and remediation program by his clinical development coach and student affairs dean because of concerns expressed by supervising faculty and residents in clerkship and post-clerkship evaluations. Although Alvarez was thought to be patient-centered and compassionate, with thorough documentation, he struggled with oral presentations, and evaluators used terms/phrases such as "disorganized," "scattered," and "includes extraneous information." His history taking did not appear to have a logical flow, and he "asked questions in no particular order as things popped into his head." Alvarez's medical knowledge, as assessed by prior standardized test scores and pre-clerkship grades, was slightly above average. He had good organizational systems for completing his daily work. He was enjoying medical school, hoping to match into a competitive residency, and denied any concerns related to mental well-being. There were no concerns related to professionalism.

REMEDIATION APPROACH

The author of this case, whom we will call Dr. Bader, worked with Alvarez as his primary clinical reasoning coach. They met 5 times (60 minutes each) over a period of 2 months, one-on-one, in person, in Dr. Bader's office. Dr. Bader spent 10 hours preparing for coaching sessions and obtaining ongoing evaluation and feedback.

> *Editor: While it may be unfair to compare two cases, the editor wants to highlight the time difference that it took to remediate a medical student who struggles with clinical reasoning (5 hours) versus a resident (11 hours). With this deficit in particular, it is crucial for the learner to develop a method of organizing their knowledge as early in training as possible. Build the scaffold while you know a little, then add to it, rather than having to go back and reassemble everything that you know. Imagine you are given a 1000-piece puzzle of the beach. It is much easier to assemble the puzzle if you are given the border pieces first, then the sky, then the water, and then the sand. If you are given all the pieces at once, it is much more difficult to sift through them to find which ones go together.*

Alvarez and Dr. Bader opened with a discussion of learner expectations and goals, including a self-assessment of Alvarez's strengths and weaknesses. They then reviewed key clinical reasoning concepts and terminology. Alvarez had learned some of these concepts during his pre-clerkship clinical skills course but, admittedly, never appreciated their importance. Dr. Bader then introduced the clinical reasoning pathway, a linear stepwise progression of diagnostic and management reasoning processes: hypothesis generation, data collection, problem representation, refinement of hypotheses, development of a working diagnosis (script selection), and management. Though the simplicity and linear nature of this pathway is not completely realistic, this process allowed the coach to identify specific deficits amenable to targeted intervention. Alvarez was asked to methodically work through cases in this stepwise fashion, with repeated prompting from Dr. Bader to think aloud. This process revealed that Alvarez especially struggled with refinement of hypotheses.

> *Editor: Many schools do not teach clinical reasoning. Students are taught clinical information in the classroom but are expected to learn clinical reasoning via the hidden curriculum either in small groups during the pre-clinical years or not until they are immersed in the clinical environment.*

It is just assumed that they will pick up this skill by watching others present on rounds and listening to their faculty think out loud. Struggling learners rarely learn from the hidden curriculum. They are still teachable; they just need to be taught more directly.[1]

Specifically, Alvarez's knowledge base allowed him to generate a broad differential based on limited clinical information. He was also able to take a complete, extremely thorough history. However, he struggled to refine his initially broad list of hypotheses into a narrow, patient-specific differential diagnosis once he gathered relevant data. To address this struggle, he was asked to work on the following exercises, applying each to a broad range of cases.

Play the Role: Assuming the role of a patient, Alvarez was asked to describe how he would convince a fictional clinician (coach) of a specific diagnosis to force prioritization of clinical details. For instance, if given a diagnosis of brain tumor or the syndrome of increased intracranial pressure, Alvarez would need to describe new onset or worsening headaches, vision changes, and morning nausea and vomiting, perhaps with a family history of malignancy – but without extraneous clinical details.

Editor: While learners often dread role play, they can find it very helpful once they get past the initial moments of self-consciousness.[2,3] *This exercise can even be framed as a game. See if you can get me to guess the diagnosis with 4 symptoms, 3 physical exams findings. (Game night at my house, anyone?)*

Assess for Fit: After obtaining a working diagnosis, Alvarez was asked to list aspects of the patient presentation that were concordant, discordant, and expected but missing for the leading diagnoses as part of a structured reflection.

It has been observed that students and trainees that struggle with clinical reasoning commonly also struggle to tolerate uncertainty, an inherent component of medicine that manifests in both diagnostic and management decision-making. This drive for certainty is a well-known bias for both practicing clinicians and learners but is likely augmented by diagnosis-focused didactic sessions and limited explicit teaching on the concept of uncertainty and its role in clinical reasoning across the spectrum of medical education.

Yet, Alvarez was different. He was exceedingly comfortable with uncertainty to the point of rigidity. In fact, in early coaching sessions, he adamantly refused to choose a working diagnosis. He described a fear of anchoring, of narrowing too early. He stated that he felt "all information the patient provided was important and should not be disregarded." Alvarez and Dr. Bader had multiple in-depth conversations about the role of a clinician, emphasizing that patient-centered care requires proper acknowledgement of all patient data, especially identification and thoughtful consideration of patient distress. However, this approach should augment, not limit, clinical reasoning. In Dr. Bader's determination, this instinct was part personality trait and part an inability to decipher relevant clinical information versus less relevant information. This was reinforced by Alvarez's evaluation data from direct observations on the wards. These evaluations described Alvarez's interview style as detailed and comprehensive, but sometimes lacking direction and organization. During coaching sessions, this disorganized data collection led to long, disorganized presentations, lengthy problem representations, and again, an inability to select a working diagnosis.

To improve this, Dr. Bader and Alvarez focused on hypothesis-driven data collection. They practiced a script search exercise during each case. For each specific chief complaint, Alvarez was asked to generate a broad differential diagnosis, then prompted to gather only 5 history items and 3 physical exam findings. This exercise forced him to consider differentiating and distinguishing features of each diagnosis. Dr. Bader then asked Alvarez to compare and contrast key features of each diagnosis. This exercise was repeated for multiple chief complaints. Alvarez was encouraged to use evidence-based medicine resources to collect information on likelihood ratios for both pertinent positives and pertinent negatives.

Next, they practiced an exercise Dr. Bader refers to as advanced problem representation. In this exercise, Alvarez was asked to write a "textbook" problem representation for a given diagnosis, preferably a diagnosis commonly encountered in clinical practice, as if he was 100% sure of the given diagnosis. Next, he was asked to consider one or two closely related diagnoses, those that might be on the differential for the proposed patient. Finally, Alvarez was required to adapt his initial problem representation to convey a greater level of uncertainty, as if he had narrowed down his differential to these two or three diagnoses instead of the initial one. This usually required inclusion of additional pertinent positives or negatives into the problem representation. This exercise prompted explicit consideration of diagnostic uncertainty as well as consideration of how uncertainty is communicated to other members of the care team. It also forced Alvarez to think of diagnoses in groups, for sake of comparison, instead of in isolation.

Editor: The benefit of ongoing development of expertise in your remediation faculty is that they can adapt their teaching strategies to the needs of the learner as Dr. Bader did in this case. An experienced teacher will know how to provide incrementally more challenging cases and appropriately disruptive questioning and take a dialogic stance that encourages more collaborative discussion. Experienced teachers are better at diagnosing cognitive errors, reviewing metacognition, and making links between the learner's cognitive patterns, knowledge, and the case at hand.[4,5]

DISCIPLINARY ACTION

None. Referral to our program is a pre-disciplinary process.

SUCCESSES

The program was successful, and Alvarez went on to do relatively well in medical school and ultimately matched into the residency of his choosing.

HINDSIGHT REFLECTIONS FROM THE REMEDIATING FACULTY

In hindsight, we wish we had begun coaching earlier, perhaps prior to Alvarez beginning clerkship. On review, although Alvarez did well academically, his pre-clerkship clinical evaluations revealed signs of future struggle. His medical knowledge and above-average test-taking ability overshadowed his struggle with application of knowledge. Earlier coaching could have provided Alvarez with a standardized framework with which to approach every patient interaction. ⌘

REFERENCES

1   Guerrasio J. *Remediation of the Struggling Medical Learner, 2nd Ed.* Irwin, PA: Association for Hospital Medical Education; 2017.

2   Deveugele M, Derese A, De Maesschalck S, Willems S, Van Driel M, De Maeseneer J. Teaching communication skills to medical students, a challenge in the curriculum? *Pat Educ and Counsel.* 2005 Sep 1;58(3):265-70.

3   Chou CL, Kalet A, Costa MJ, et al. Guidelines: The dos, don'ts and don't knows of remediation in medical education. *Perspect Med Educ.* 2019;8:322-338.

4   Winston K. Cees PM, van der Vleuten AJJ, Scherpbier A. Core concepts in remediation: Lessons learned from a 6-year case study. *Med Sci Educ.* 2105 June;(25)307-315.

5   Winston KA, van der Vleuten CP, Scherpbier AJ. Prediction and prevention of failure: An early intervention to assist at-risk medical students. *Med Teach.* 2014 Jan 1;36(1):25-31.

CASE 14

Medical Knowledge and Time Management and Organization

LEARNER AT TIME OF IDENTIFICATION FOR REMEDIATION

Michelle, a third-year physician assistant student

REASON FOR REMEDIATION

Phase 1 – Informal Remediation

At the conclusion of the didactic phase of physician assistant (PA) training, students complete a formative clinical assessment that involves 4 standardized patient cases. Students are assessed on communication skills, physical examination performance, and an oral or written post-encounter activity for each clinical case. The results from this assessment showed that Michelle was at least 1 standard deviation below the mean in 1 or more task areas for all 4 clinical cases. On 3 of the 4 cases, Michelle scored 1 to 2 standard deviations below the mean for the overall case score. For the total evaluation score, she scored 2 standard deviations below the mean.

Because this assessment was considered formative, the faculty felt that Michelle could benefit from informal remediation. Per the institution's student academic policies and procedures, only a failed evaluation, rather than a formative assessment, can warrant formal remediation and halt progress to the clinical year. Therefore, Michelle was offered and accepted an informal remediation plan created and instituted by the informal remediation team, which consisted of 3 core faculty members.

Editor: The concept of informal versus formal remediation is very confusing to struggling learners and general teaching faculty alike. What are the differences? Will the learner see informal remediation more like suggestions rather than strategies that they must try to implement? When the learner is asked if they have been on remediation, is one reportable and the other not? Should one be taken more seriously by the learner than the other? Do general teaching faculty need to participate in informal remediation or does the informality make it optional?

If remediation is separated from disciplinary action, there is no need for it to be declared formal or informal. Remediation can stand alone and be available to anyone who needs it. Warning or probation are disciplinary actions; they are formal. Disciplinary action plans can stipulate remediation without having to label remediation as formal or otherwise.

REMEDIATION APPROACH

1. The informal remediation team gathered holistic information on Michelle including admission information, didactic and clinical course grades and feedback, prior formative clinical assessment reports, and formative written assessment reports – including a PACKRAT score of 102 out of 225 (below passing) – to identify her areas of deficiency. The areas of deficiency identified were medical knowledge and time management and organization, specifically with SOAP note writing and oral presentations.

   *Editor: The PACKRAT is a national formative comprehensive written assessment given periodically in PA school to assess student progress. It is a multiple-choice question test. PACKRAT stands for **p**hysician **a**ssistant **c**linical **k**nowledge **r**ating and **a**ssessment **t**ool.*

2. As Michelle began her clinical year, her remediation plan included being assigned tasks that targeted the identified areas of weakness – in addition to completing her clinical rotations. The tasks were as follows:

    a. Create a table to organize her cognitive process for each topic missed on the exam. The informal remediation team called this her "cognitive organizer."

    b. Meet with the informal remediation team every two weeks to review the tables and orally present a patient from her clinical rotation that month using the SOAP note format

    c. Complete weekly medical knowledge quiz questions using the product Board Vitals®

3. Michelle's informal remediation began with the clinical year and concluded after 4 months when the team felt that she was no longer progressing based on the scores of the weekly Board Vitals® exam. Simultaneously, Michelle that she felt she no longer needed assistance.

Editor: Tables are a great way to help learners expand their knowledge base while simultaneously guiding that knowledge into scaffolds that connect pieces of their knowledge into a more cohesive picture. This cohesion then allows for diagnoses to be compared and contrasted. Such scaffolds are helpful for clinical reasoning when learners are presented with symptoms rather than diagnoses and have to decide, for example, if the wheezing patient has asthma or chronic obstructive lung disease.[1,2]

    It is unclear why the remediation team stopped when Michelle's progress halted. While underperforming learners can often identify their areas of weakness, they are notoriously bad at determining their level of competence.[3,4] *Remediation should continue until the learner is able to demonstrate that they have gained the previously insufficient skills, or it is determined that the goals cannot be met within the given time frame and available resources of the training program.*

    In this case, a proper assessment is warranted to evaluate medical knowledge and time management and organization before remediation is declared complete. For medical knowledge, an exam can be given.[5] *To assess time management and organization for her, consider having 3 independent faculty complete a mini CEX (observed clinical examine) complete with SOAP notes and presentation.*

Two months after the informal remediation plan, Michelle received below-average scores in multiple competencies on a required clinical rotation evaluation. The areas that were marked as below average included medical knowledge, history-taking, physical exam skills, medical decision-making, creation of a plan, SOAP note generation, time management, ability to identify gaps in knowledge, and interpersonal and communication skills. These deficiencies equated to below-average performance in 5 of the 6 competencies assessed: medical knowledge, patient care, practice-based learning and improvement, interpersonal and communication skills, and systems-based practice. Based on this evaluation and the comments provided from multiple preceptors at the clinical site, the student was determined to have failed this clinical rotation. Based on the student academic policies and procedures, due to the failure, Michelle was placed on academic probation and provided with a formal remediation team to create a formal remediation plan.

Phase 2 – Formal Remediation

The formal remediation team consisted of 3 core faculty members that were neither on Michelle's informal remediation team nor served as her academic advisors.

1. The formal remediation team began by gathering and reviewing holistic data on Michelle including all the data obtained by the informal remediation team, subsequent data and communications that occurred during the informal remediation plan, and clinical rotation evaluation data including the failed rotation evaluation.

   Editor: This illustrates another reason why having an informal and formal remediation process is suboptimal. It is extremely disruptive to the process. Why are new faculty having to learn who this student is and develop a new relationship with her? Bonds of trust are essential to the remediation process. This change will sever any bonds that have developed.[6,7] It is unlikely that a second set of eyes is going to see the challenges differently. If the first team needs help, they can always discuss their challenges with other education faculty, gather their suggestions, then bring any feasible ideas back to the learner. Also, faculty time is valuable (and expensive). The redundancy of effort seems like time that could be better spent working with the learner in need.

2. Using the same approach as the informal remediation team, the remediation framework provided in the book *Remediation of the Struggling Medical Learner* was used to categorize the student's deficits. Although Michelle had multiple deficit areas, the formal remediation team felt that the two most significant areas of deficit were (1) medical knowledge and (2) time management and organization. These were the same deficit areas identified in the original informal remediation plan.

3. Approximately 10 days after the conclusion of the failed rotation, the chair met with Michelle to gather her perspective on her deficits. The following questions were asked regarding her medical knowledge deficit:

   • What does Michelle identify as her deficits?
   • What has she been doing to help her medical knowledge deficit?
   • What barriers did she experience with the informal remediation plan?
   • What barriers does she believe she may encounter now?

Editor: These are great check-in questions, especially if they can be asked by someone that the learner trusts. It will be helpful to know if she agrees with the faculty's assessment of her. What does she know about her learning history that her faculty may not know? Perhaps she will reveal a prior learning disorder or previous learning challenge. What is working for her? What is not working for her? Not all strategies work for everyone. Learners should be encouraged to try new strategies with the caveat that everyone is different, so if one of the strategies doesn't work, it can be replaced with another – but suggestions should at least be given a fair chance. Unforeseen barriers are common, and plans need to be fluid. Further, not all rotations or faculty are as the remediation team might anticipate. Asking about limitations to implementing the plan will help both Michelle and the team.

4. The following questions were asked of Michelle regarding the time management and organization deficit:

   • Is this a new problem? Does this also exist outside of school?
   • What strategies has she used in her personal life to prepare and stay organized?
   • What has she tried to improve this deficit?
   • Has she been using the cognitive organizer and templates provided to her by the informal remediation team?

   Editor: Most challenges are not new to the learner. Many of our learners are so bright that they have been able to compensate for their deficits until faced with the great challenges that medical professional schools demand. Others need to be reminded of learning strategies that worked well in the past that they may have abandoned, or that need to be adapted to this new learning environment. If a learner sees that their struggles are not unique to school or residency, they will be more willing to own the deficit and to seek help.

   Some people manage their time best by making a list, while others do best by setting time limits for activities. There are many different strategies for time management and organization. Your learner will likely need to try out a few before they find what works for them. Many faculty think their way is the only and best way, and it is – but only for them and others like them. This is one area where it is helpful to find others who have overcome similar struggles and utilize their input when building the remediation plan.[8]

5. Following the interview process, the formal remediation plan was presented to Michelle. The goal for the formal remediation plan was the implementation and completion of a focused, intensive remediation plan occurring over 3 months, then 2 months of faculty-guided remediation followed by 1 month of student self-directed learning to prepare for the final assessments. Michelle would be removed from

clinical rotations during this time to focus on her remediation plan. Each member of the remediation team was actively involved in the weekly sessions with Michelle, grading of materials (SOAP notes and oral presentations) based on established validated rubrics, monthly team meetings, and the final recommendations at the conclusion of the remediation plan provided to the student promotions committee.

The remediation team felt strongly that Michelle's ability to return to clinic rotations was dependent on her progress in the benchmark areas established by the remediation team. The benchmarks for progress were (1) receiving a score of at least 70% on the weekly Board Vitals multiple-choice exams, (2) completion of her cognitive organizer based on weekly clinical cases, and (3) weekly case presentations of at least "meets expectations" on all 4 domains in an oral presentation and SOAP note rubric. The clinical cases would cover clinical presentations and medical topics found within all body systems. The final assessments to determine completion of the formal remediation were based on successful completion of the clinical year assessment with 8 standardized patient cases and retaking the formative written assessment (PACKRAT) with a satisfactory assessment score.

In addition to the plans and schedules, the remediation team encouraged Michelle to engage in the following learning and self-care activities:

- understand why and when, rather than how or what to do next
- compare and contrast diseases with similar presentations
- link reading to patient cases
- limit caffeine
- get 6 hours of sleep per night
- identify when she studies best during the day
- consider external resources for needs (office of disabilities and resource services, office of case management services)
- identify stress management strategies
- seek evaluation from an outside professional service

The medical knowledge and time management and organization plans, faculty schedule, and student schedule are provided below. (See **Tables 14.1-4**)

TABLE 14.1 Medical Knowledge Plan

Item	Quantity	Due Date	Score Goal	Other
Board vitals exams	Daily = 100 questions/day; total = 500 questions/week	Weekly = every Friday by 12 PM	70%	Review scores with faculty member
Cognitive organizer	Notify team if completing as a Google spreadsheet or in a notebook	Weekly = reviewed by remediation team every Friday		Access from student provided to remediation team for weekly review
PACKRAT – written assessment	225 Questions	Final Assessment	120	Goal = end of 2-month remediation

TABLE 14.2 Time Management and Organization Plan

Item	Quantity	Due Date	Score Goal	Other
Oral presentation of patient case: organization of patient visit – integrating medical knowledge and patient care	2 cases/week	Weekly – Fridays	70% correct	Provide H&P template. Given a patient's age, sex, and CC, student will elicit a patient history, explain the components of the physical exam pertinent to the patient's problem, provide an assessment with 3 top diagnoses and medical decision making, and generate a plan with patient education.
SOAP note documentation of patient case: organization of patient visit – integrating medical knowledge and patient care	2 cases/week – discussed on Friday	Weekly – Monday following case discussion that occurred on prior Friday	70% correct	All components of the case are organized, succinct, and accurate based on the patient case. Submit via a Word document to allow for track changes.
Clinical year clinical exam	Final assessment		Pass	Goal = end of 2-month remediation

TABLE 14.3 Faculty Remediation Schedule

Week	Monday	Friday	Following Monday	Faculty Assigned	Block
Week #1	Send student age, sex and CC ONLY for 2 cases	Pull board review scores after 12 PM Review cognitive organizer completion Meet with student to complete 2 cases Score rubrics	Grade 2 SOAP notes from weekly cases	#1	Summer
Week #2	Send student age, sex and CC ONLY for 2 cases	Pull board review scores after 12 PM Review cognitive organizer completion Meet with student to complete 2 cases Score rubrics	Grade 2 SOAP notes from weekly cases	#2	Hematology, immunology, infection, and malignancy
Week #3	Send student age, sex and CC ONLY for 2 cases	Pull board review scores after 12 PM Review cognitive organizer completion Meet with student to complete 2 cases Score rubrics	Grade 2 SOAP notes from weekly cases	#3	Gastrointestinal, genitourinary, renal
Week #4	Send student age, sex and CC ONLY for 2 cases	Pull board review scores after 12 PM Review cognitive organizer completion Meet with student to complete 2 cases Score rubrics	Grade 2 SOAP notes from weekly cases	#3	Endocrinology, reproduction

TABLE 14.3 Faculty Remediation Schedule *(cont'd)*

Week	Monday	Friday	Following Monday	Faculty Assigned	Block
Week #5	Send student age, sex and CC ONLY for 2 cases	Pull board review scores after 12 PM Review cognitive organizer completion Meet with student to complete 2 cases Score rubrics	Grade 2 SOAP notes from weekly cases	#2	Dermatology, HEENT
Week #6	Send student age, sex and CC ONLY for 2 cases	Pull board review scores after 12 PM Review cognitive organizer completion Meet with student to complete 2 cases Score rubrics	Grade 2 SOAP notes from weekly cases	#1	Musculoskeletal, neurology
Week #7	Send student age, sex and CC ONLY for 2 cases	Pull board review scores after 12 PM Review cognitive organizer completion Meet with student to complete 2 cases Score rubrics	Grade 2 SOAP notes from weekly cases	#3	Psychiatry
Week #8	Send student age, sex and CC ONLY for 2 cases	Pull PACKRAT scores after 12 PM Review cognitive organizer completion Meet with student to complete 2 cases Score rubrics	Grade 2 SOAP notes from weekly cases	#1	Cardiovascular, pulmonary

TABLE 14.4 **Student Remediation Schedule**

Week	Mon	Tues	Wed	Thu	Fri	Faculty
Week #1–6	2 cases provided for the week – review for Friday	Board vitals Cognitive organizer H&P templates	Board vitals Cognitive organizer H&P templates	Board vitals Cognitive organizer H&P templates	500 board vitals questions completed by 12 PM Completed cognitive organizers with access to faculty 2 cases with faculty member completed Friday afternoon	#1, #2 or #3
Week #7		Remediation team to present findings and rec-ommendations to student promotions team				
Week #8	PACKRAT 2 cases provided for the week – review for Friday 2 SOAP notes due at 12 PM from Friday cases	PACKRAT Cognitive organizer H&P templates	PACKRAT Cognitive organizer H&P templates	PACKRAT completed by 12 PM Cognitive organizer H&P templates	Completed cognitive organizers with access to faculty 2 cases with faculty member completed Friday afternoon	#1, #2 or #3
Final Month				Clinical year clinical exam	Clinical year clinical exam	

DISCIPLINARY ACTION

In this PA program, the Student Promotions Committee "may impose academic probation in instances of unsatisfactory grades or unprofessional behavior. The length of probation is determined on a case-by-case basis but may continue until graduation." Due to the initial course failure, Michelle was placed on academic probation. When a student is placed on academic probation, the student is automatically referred to the university's Office of Case Management. The Office of Case Management serves as an advocate and guide to the student towards additional resources and services the student may need (e.g., mental health services, office of disability and resource services, healthcare services, etc.)

> *Editor: Remember, professionalism is also an academic competency. Had her issue been professionalism, she should have been placed on academic probation as well. The editor wants to make a tangential point not to separate professionalism from any other academic competency, as you could legally open the institution up to interference from the courts. The judicial system will defer to academic institutions regarding academic decisions; since professionalism is an academic competency, do not separate it from the other academic competencies.*

The University's legal department was consulted throughout the duration of the remediation plan, as they have years of experience at the institution and are tremendously helpful and supportive. Their motto is "Do the right thing for the learner **and** society, and we will support you." Because of concerns around possible external factors contributing to the student's struggles, Michelle was mandated to seek an evaluation by the state's Physician Health Program, which provides comprehensive health and wellness evaluations for physician assistants as well as physicians. Given the length of the remediation plan, she successfully graduated but her graduation was delayed.

OPPORTUNITIES TO LEARN

The informal remediation plan did not work well primarily because this was a voluntary plan provided to the student based on concerning performance that had not yet progressed to a failure of a course or clinical rotation. Unfortunately, because there were no mandated requirements in place for the informal remediation plan, the student had self-imposed flexibility on how and when she completed specific tasks. This created a significant amount of work for the informal remediation team who created activities for the student with regular check-ins, only to find that the remediation plan was not a top priority for the student. The student was also allowed to continue her clinical rotations during the informal remediation and noted that time constraints and demands from her clinical rotation prevented her from achieving the suggested benchmarks.

In contrast, the formal remediation plan with concrete required benchmarks, timelines, and outcomes worked better for this student. Working with three faculty on a weekly basis, with standardized rubrics and final assessments, allowed for an objective measure of the student's progress and achievement of outcomes. The student and the faculty were able to assess progress and provide feedback and correction immediately using the timelines and benchmarks as references. ⌇

REFERENCES

1   Guerrasio J, Aagaard EM. Methods and outcomes for the remediation of clinical reasoning. *JGIM*. 2014 Dec 1;29(12):1607-14.

2   De Grave WS, Dolmans DH, van der Vleuten CP. Profiles of effective tutors in problem based learning: scaffolding student learning. *Med Educ*. 1999 Dec;33(12):901-6.

3   Patel R, Tarrant C, Bonas S, Yates J, Sandars J. The struggling student: a thematic analysis from the self-regulated learning perspective. *Med Educ*. 2015;49:417-26.

4   Kruger J, Dunning D. Unskilled and unaware of it: how difficulties in recognizing one's own incompetence lead to inflated self-assessments. *J Pers Soc Psychol*. 1999;77:1121-34.

5   Hawthorne MR, Chretien KC, Torre D, Chheda SG. Redemonstration without remediation – a missed opportunity? A national survey of internal medicine clerkship directors. *Med Educ Online*. 2014;19:25991.

6   Kalet A, Chou CL, Ellaway RH. To fail is human: remediating remediation in medical education. *Perspect Med Educ*. 2017;6:418-24.

7   Bennion LD, Durning SJ, LaRochelle J, et al. Untying the Gordian knot: remediation problems in medical schools that need remediation. *BMC Med Educ*. 2018;18:120.

8   Guerrasio J. *Remediation of the Struggling Medical Learner, 2nd Ed*. Irwin, PA: Association for Hospital Medical Education; 2017.

Clinical Reasoning, Time Management and Organization, Clinical Skills, Interpersonal Skills, and Mental Well-Being

LEARNER AT TIME OF IDENTIFICATION FOR REMEDIATION

Will, a second-year optometry student starting clinical rotations

REASON FOR REMEDIATION

Even though Will had received his bachelor's degree from a prestigious undergraduate college, he still struggled in optometry school.

Editor: While many students get a more rigorous education at higher-rated undergraduate institutions, there are no guarantees that they will be successful in professional school. For example, undergraduate education doesn't usually assess professionalism, communication skills, interpersonal skills, or manual dexterity. An applicant's competence in these areas is largely unknown. Perhaps group projects in addition to multiple mini-interviews on interview day could help elucidate some of these characteristics.[1]

The assessment and evaluation of a student's knowledge attainment and problem-solving skills depends on a student's major and the amount of support that they may have received during their undergraduate education. Some support improves students' ability to learn and to be self-driven learners and helps them become better professional school candidates. Others receive support (e.g., note takers, heavy reliance on tutors, ability to avoid courses that require reading, small or easy course loads, extra time to complete assignments, therapy pets, etc.) that cannot be replicated in a clinical environment. This puts these students at a disadvantage when compared with their peers.

The editor has noticed over the past 15 years that students are receiving increasing amounts of external supports and mental health support to succeed in undergraduate coursework. Although the editor supports both, this results in inconsistent validation of skills upon graduation. As a result, more students are requiring remediation upon entering professional school than in the past. It is increasingly common for students to lack strong educational foundations, be short on disciplined and effective study skills and habits, and have insufficient coping mechanisms for anxiety and overcoming adversity. As for the clinical environment, previously accommodated educational support services may no longer work due to patient safety concerns. This requires remediation faculty to find new tools and strategies that will work and can be implemented for individual learners.

Will's difficulties were recognized in the clinical optometry course which includes both didactic course work and practice labs. He was identified for remediation due to challenges with clinical skills and a scattered thought process that led to insufficient time management. In the practice labs, Will and his peers were taught physical exam skills to detect eye abnormalities and to make diagnoses. The lab course requires not only motor skills, but also a level of processing to determine one's exam flow to properly and efficiently diagnose patients.

Will had passed the first-year courses but was failing the assessments in the second-year laboratories. This included testing with the slit lamp, measuring intraocular pressures, and a dilated fundus examination. He exhibited a tremor that he attributed to anti-psychotic-medication. This made it more difficult for tasks such as holding a lens steady when assessing the retina in a slit lamp or in free space. Due to the difficulty completing basic testing, the results would often be incorrect – which secondarily made analyzing data more difficult. Mini-tests throughout the semester require students to think about "next logical steps" as if they were examining a real patient. Will never seemed to absorb the reasoning for the ordering of tests and always seemed to be visually searching for the next logical task.

REMEDIATION APPROACH

After his first two semesters, Will wasn't really on the radar as he had a GPA over 3.0 and seemed to be doing average overall. He then failed a course and the associated lab assessments. At that point he was immediately matched with an advisor for the didactic portion of the course and a coach for the clinical skill set needed to continue with his training. Dr. Pete, acting as his coach, met with Will almost weekly for 6 months, checking in with his academic advisor occasionally to make sure Will was staying afloat with his study schedule.

Editor: The faculty clearly showed their dedication in the abundant amount of time they spent with Will. What is not clear is what they did with this time. It may be that they used the time very effectively but had a learner who wasn't teachable or willing to be taught. My sense is that Will was one of the rare students that fall into the "not teachable" category.[2] However, I want to point out that most mentors take an ad hoc, unstructured approach to remediation – which invariably fails. Decades of research on struggling learners has shown that unstructured mentor meetings don't improve learner competence.

When the remediation team implements a plan, it doesn't always succeed on the first attempt. If it doesn't succeed, yet the learner is invested and trying, first revisit the diagnosis of the learner's deficits. If the diagnosis is accurate and the remediation plan is designed to target that key deficit, then consider neuropsychiatric testing.[2] The learner may have an undiagnosed learning disorder or other disorder that is preventing them from learning. Perhaps there is either a treatable diagnosis or some additional information that could guide the remediation team on how to best teach this learner. In this case specifically, it is unclear why he was on an anti-psychotic and if additional neuropsychiatric testing may have helped his personal doctor modify his treatment plan to eliminate the medication which was causing disruptive side effects.

DISCIPLINARY ACTION

After receiving failing grades in two different courses in the fall semester of his second year, Will was placed on academic probation and enrolled in the academic advising. Given the choice, he repeated the second-year curriculum the following year. Having failed his second attempt, Will was dismissed from the program.

Editor: When a student learner is failing, repeating curriculum is an option to consider. It may be required based on your institution's policies and procedures. Unfortunately, this student accrued an additional year of debt before leaving with neither a degree nor a career. His lack of manual dexterity made success in his chosen career very limited, although he could potentially have gone on to teach, speak, write, or do research in optometry. Students sometimes have trouble acknowledging that they are likely to fail out of school and need the help of faculty to minimize the damages and help them with career counseling.[3]

SUCCESSES

Repetition seemed to be a great tool to help Will during his time at school. "Drills" were run for many weeks to make sure that he was comfortable with the basic skills and could figure out how to troubleshoot problems if something went wrong. He did show improvement, and his confidence also seemed to improve.

Illness scripts were used to help organize Will's thoughts when classifying diseases. Role playing helped when working in scenarios for case history practice runs. Will also found that working with an upperclassman helped him learn a few tricks to make some skills easier. In terms of organization during the lab, he found that physically organizing the materials helped him to predict the exam flow and what test he should do next.

OPPORTUNITIES TO LEARN

The "timed drills" did have a drawback: they seemed to induce stress and led to some discouraging breakdowns.

In the end, all these tools were not enough to help Will. In spite of the fact that he was motivated to put in the time and effort to do the work, self-assessment remained a weakness. He continued to get flustered during timed assessments which caused him to spiral into failure.

Editor: In reading the words, "Self-assessment remained a weakness," the first translation is "He had little to no insight." Struggling learners do very often struggle with insight.[4,5] *Why? They have trouble seeing and receiving feedback. But consider, how would I have known to speak up louder when I teach if a person in the back row hadn't told me they couldn't hear me? I recognized that as feedback and have since changed my behavior by either speaking louder or asking for a microphone. Now I know that I have a quiet voice. Feedback is essential to having insight! If you think your learner has no insight, work with them on learning how to ask for and receive feedback.*

HINDSIGHT REFLECTIONS FROM THE REMEDIATING FACULTY

Will acknowledged having a learning disability (now referred to as a learning disorder). If we had addressed his learning disorder earlier, perhaps it would have changed the outcome.

Editor: Once he had failed, perhaps the promotions committee could have mandated an independent party to conduct a physical and mental health evaluation to see that he was getting the most appropriate treatment. At the very least, his medications were interfering with his manual dexterity. Maybe there were other possible treatment options.

Most students don't know that there are technical standards that must be met for each professional school, and while disabilities can be accommodated, the standards still need to be met for the sake of patient safety. 💬

REFERENCES

1   Eva KW, Rosenfeld J, Reiter HI, Norman GR. An admissions OSCE: the multiple mini-interview. *Med Educ.* 2004; 38(3):314-26.

2   Guerrasio J. "The Prognosis is poor:" When to give up. In: Kalet A, Chou CL, editors. *Remediation in Medical Education: A mid-course correction.* Heidelberg, Berlin, New York: Springer;2014.

3   Kalet A, Chou CL, Ellaway RH. To fail is human: remediating remediation in medical education. *Perspect Med Educ.* 2017;6:418-24.

4   Cleland J, Arnold R, Chessar A. Failing finals is often a surprise for the student but not the teacher: identifying difficulties and supporting students with academic difficulties. *Med Teach* 2005;27(6):504-8.

5   Hodges B, Regehr G, Martin D. Difficulties in recognizing one's own incompetence: novice physicians who are unskilled and unaware of it. *Acad Med.* 2001 Oct 1;76(10):S87-9.

CASE 16

Time Management and Organization, Communication, Clinical Reasoning, and Professionalism

LEARNER AT TIME OF IDENTIFICATION FOR REMEDIATION

Lisa, a third-year optometry student

REASON FOR REMEDIATION

While having a great bedside manner is admirable, it becomes a problem when it affects one's ability to be productive. Efficiency was an issue for Lisa, who really enjoyed conversing with her patients.

> *Editor: Time management is another skill that students need to learn to be successful in clinical medicine. Sometimes learners place a clock in the room where they can easily see it, but the patient cannot. Other learners prefer to set a timer for themselves with an audible or vibrating alarm that alerts them to move on to the next part of the encounter. Perhaps the most helpful method is to have a plan for the patient encounter before you walk into the room. Why is the patient here? What is the clinical setting? Is it an emergency? Is it a new patient, new problem, or follow-up visit? Having an agenda for the encounter before walking into the room helps with time management, organization, and efficiency and hones clinical reasoning.*[1]

Next, Lisa's scattered presentations led her supervisors to question her background knowledge. Her ability to multitask and analyze data in real time were also suboptimal. All of these things considered, it was her inability to self-reflect that truly limited her ability to succeed.

From her perspective, Lisa felt she was doing well and seemed rather surprised by her sub-par midterm clinical grades. She continued to struggle to incorporate weekly feedback. She needed remediation for time management and organization, communication, clinical reasoning, and professionalism due to her denial and poor self-reflection.

> *Editor: For some disciplines, denial of feedback, educational challenges, and poor self-reflection would fall under the category of problem-based learning and improvement. However, considering Lisa's specific reaction, evoking unprofessional behavior may also fall under poor professionalism. The deficit categories certainly have some areas where they overlap.*[2]

REMEDIATION APPROACH

The remediation process began with a review of the weekly feedback comments from Lisa's current clinical attendings. Dr. Harris, her remediation coach, shadowed her during live encounters in the clinic to observe her physical assessment skills, diagnostic thought processes, and ability to communicate efficiently with her patients and attendings. Dr. Harris later assessed each encounter and had Lisa reflect on what went well and on what points she felt she could improve. Lisa and Dr. Harris also continued working outside the clinic by using role playing to practice efficient and complete history intake.

> *Editor: This remediation plan is full of direct observation and role playing, with feedback and reflection on how to change her practice and performance. The active nature of this plan increases its likelihood of success.*[3]

During the time of clinical remediation, Lisa began studying for the national board examination. This, in turn, helped improve her clinical analysis skills as her medical knowledge solidified. Lisa met with Dr. Harris every two weeks for about four months. As her clinical grades improved, they met less frequently. Dr. Harris made 3 final monthly checks on Lisa to ensure she continued to progress.

Editor: Lisa actually possessed the ability to clinically analyze patient information, but prior to having sufficient knowledge, this skill was untested. Sometimes when medical knowledge is remediated, the ability to clinical reason is found to be intact. Other times it reveals another deficit that needs remediation.

DISCIPLINARY ACTION

No disciplinary actions were taken.

SUCCESSES

Dr. Harris believed that the most beneficial practices were repeatedly reviewing cases that Lisa had seen in the clinic and role-playing. As Lisa learned to go through an exam sequence more logically in her head, her organization improved. She was able to concisely present a case to her supervisors with a more solid analysis of each case. This gave her more confidence. Lisa's self-awareness in clinic improved. She was gradually able to understand what she wasn't comfortable with in clinic and how to improve by using feedback effectively. Once Lisa's basic skills became easier, she was better able to multitask and speak to patients while completing tasks, e.g., cleaning equipment or setting up the next test. She successfully moved forward and reached full levels of competency.

Editor: Not every learner will graduate in the top half of their class. But every graduate needs to know what they know and what they don't know, when to ask for help, and have the humility to do so. Not only did Lisa's skills improve, but there is a sense of reassurance that she's safe to practice.

Ultimately, every institution which graduates learners has a societal and ethical obligation to ensure that its graduates can fulfill their professional role responsibly and safely, providing high-quality and professional care. If learners know when to ask for help and understand the boundaries of their abilities to practice, this will assure those granting qualifications that they are ready to be independent.[4]

REFERENCES

1   Guerrasio J. *Remediation of the Struggling Medical Learner, 2nd Ed.* Irwin, PA: Association for Hospital Medical Education; 2017.

2   Carraccio C, Wolfsthal SD, Englander R, Ferentz K, Martin C. Shifting paradigms: from Flexner to competencies. *Acad Med.* 2002 May 1;77(5):361-7.

3   Warburton KM, Goren E, Dine CJ. Comprehensive assessment of struggling learners referred to a graduate medical education remediation program. *JGME.* 2017 Dec;9(6):763-7.

4   Ellaway RH, Chou CL, Kalet AL. Situating remediation: accommodating success and failure in medical education systems. *Acad Med.* 2018;93:391-8.

CASE 17

Communication and Interpersonal Skills

LEARNER AT TIME OF IDENTIFICATION FOR REMEDIATION

José, a third-year medical student on his first core clinical clerkship

REASON FOR REMEDIATION

The original complaint against José was that he manifested unprofessional behavior during his first clinical rotation while interacting with his supervising physicians, other members of the health care team, and patients. After further investigation it was determined that José's primary deficit was not professionalism, but rather his interpersonal and communication skills.

The initial concerns revolved around José's difficulties working effectively with his supervising residents and a junior faculty attending physician on his pediatric rotation. His patient presentations were noted to be disorganized and incomplete. The senior resident on the team was asked by the attending physician to work with José to improve this skill. When the senior resident complied, José was noted to be resistant to his efforts and acted disinterested when the senior resident provided José with a handout detailing how to deliver new patient presentations and daily follow-up patient presentations using the SOAP format. José seemed to find this demeaning and stated that the senior resident and attending physician were prejudiced against him due to his Latino heritage. On teaching rounds the next day, José refused to present his assigned patients and told the attending that he did not think he was being treated fairly.

Editor: Before proceeding, it will be important to know if José's other skills are up to par. Is he behaving this way to mask other clinical performance deficits or psychological challenges related to lack of confidence? How had he performed in his first two years of medical school? Were there any previous struggles with poor professional behaviors or interpersonal skills and communication?

We know that learners with deficits will minimize their struggles and externalize by blaming faculty and the institution for their poor assessments.[1,2] When a learner feels that they are being assessed unfairly, it helps to bring in one or more unbiased third parties to conduct an independent assessment of the learner's skills. Sometimes learners actually are treated unfairly.[3] It is best practice to collect additional assessments from others who are unaware of any prior concerns. In this case, 1 or 2 faculty members can conduct an observed mini-CEX (clinical exam) with oral presentation and SOAP note to verify or refute the observations noted by the team.[4] If the observations are not verified, it could be due to the limited number of cases observed, as the deficit may be topic specific, or it may truly be an unfair original assessment. However, the deficits are almost always readily apparent.

At the same time this was occurring, José was approached by a nurse on the adolescent unit who was concerned that he was inappropriate in his communication with a pre-teen girl hospitalized on the unit for gastrointestinal issues. José had been observed siting on the edge of the patient's bed talking with her in a flirtatious manner. The nurse relayed that the patient's father had approached her and asked that José not continue to see his daughter as he felt his daughter was becoming infatuated with José. He expressed that he felt José was not acting professionally and did not seem appropriately focused on his daughter's medical concerns.

Finally, a social worker assigned to the pediatric inpatient unit stated that José was making her feel very uncomfortable as he regularly complimented her on her dress, her hair, her smile, and her perfume. She tried to deflect his attention by talking about patients they were seeing together, but José seemed disinterested in those discussions.

Editor: From the editor's experience, most institutions would remove this student from clinical rotations immediately to conduct an investigation and allow for an independent physical and mental health evaluation to ensure his fitness to care for patients ("fitness for duty evaluation"). He would otherwise need continuous supervision while in the clinical setting, which is practically unfeasible. If the reports are confirmed, disciplinary action of probation would follow.

Fitness to care for patients, also referred to as fitness for duty, is about protecting patients and the public. It is the responsibility of medical schools and medical training programs to ensure that patients are protected from harm. Fitness to practice is about minimum acceptable standards. While some professionalism violations may result in the need to assess the learner's fitness for duty, most will not.[5] In the United Kingdom, students have been declared unfit for duty for lack of insight, lack of remediation, dishonesty, and for health reasons.[6]

The attending physician called Dean Simon to report that the student was having serious professionalism issues with multiple members of the health care team and asked that the dean meet with José to discuss these concerns. When Dean Simon met with José and asked him if he knew why they were meeting, José insisted it was because the entire pediatric patient care team was prejudiced against him. José was frustrated that those members of the team who had concerns about him were telling others on the team, thereby prejudicing them against him.

An ad hoc committee was set up to investigate whether there was any implicit or explicit bias involved in the way José was being treated. Speaking with the involved parties, the committee also discussed the importance of privately addressing concerns about José and not sharing information with others beyond him and his direct supervisors. This did lead to better recognition by the pediatric care team of the challenges facing José and a shared understanding of how to help him, while assuring that he was being treated and evaluated fairly and objectively.

Dean Simon took the time to ask José how his first two years of medical school had gone. José proceeded to tell the dean that the pre-clinical years had been very difficult for him. He had done well enough academically and passed all his courses, but he had not made any friends and felt very alone. He explained that moving from a Latinx community in his home state to a small out-of-state community for medical school (where there were very few Latinx students) had not been easy. When Dean Simon asked if he had depressive symptoms, he admitted to feelings of sadness and isolation but denied any other indicators of clinical depression; he specifically denied any suicidal thoughts.

REMEDIATION APPROACH

Remediation efforts included arranging for a mental health evaluation, establishing a mentor, and providing regular coaching to improve José's communication and reporting skills. In addition, close monitoring of his performance on subsequent clinical clerkships was arranged.

> *Editor: A word of caution. If you only refer a struggling learner for a mental health evaluation, you might miss a medical problem that is impacting their performance. You could also be accused of making an assumption that the learner has a psychiatric problem, which could open the institution up to legal risk. Remember, although we are clinicians, we are not the learner's clinicians. Recommend a complete evaluation and leave it up to the learner's treating providers to help you. You can require that the struggling learner sign a release of information so that you can talk with those providers, if the learner is placed on disciplinary action.*
>
> *Even though this book spends most of its pages discussing struggling learners, patient safety is always the priority. In this case, monitoring would need to be continuous. It is easy to think of minors and those with impaired cognition as being vulnerable, but in truth all patients are vulnerable and need to be protected from students, residents, and faculty who behave unprofessionally.*

Early in their work together, Dean Simon arranged for José to be seen in the counseling center for a mental health evaluation. This proved helpful as José developed a good therapeutic relationship with one of the PhD counselors, and he continued to visit with this counselor on a monthly basis to talk through some of his feelings of isolation. The counselor did not find evidence for any substance abuse and did not feel a psychiatric evaluation or referral for medication was needed.

Dean Simon next arranged for José to meet with a young Latino physician who Dean Simon thought could be an excellent role model and mentor. Although they did not develop a mentoring relationship, it was helpful as the young physician convinced José that the concerns raised about his behavior were legitimate and needed his attention.

Editor: José had already verbalized that he felt isolated and lonely without having others from his Latinx culture and community. It is appropriate to offer assistance in connecting José to others from either the Latinx community or the underrepresented minority (URM) community. Some institutions have social or support groups and/or mentoring communities for underrepresented minorities (URMs.)

Dean Simon then observed José interview a pediatric patient newly admitted to the inpatient unit and found it very instructive. José's interview lacked organization, and he failed to address several key areas with the patient and the patient's mother. His subsequent verbal presentation was similarly disorganized. When Dean Simon shared that he was concerned about José's interview and verbal presentation skills, José became quite defensive and insisted that the patient and the patient's mother were not good historians, which made his efforts more difficult.

Dean Simon was able to convince José that his sole interest was in helping José develop his communication skills and seeing him become the best physician possible. Dean Simon asked José to write an essay about how interpersonal skills and communication with patients and their families, peers, supervising residents, attending physicians, nurses, and other members of the health care team were important to providing good patient care. When they met to discuss José's essay, they discussed how failing in any one of these areas could negatively affect assessment of José's competence and ultimately his ability to achieve his dream of becoming a physician.

Editor: As the remediation plan progresses, we can see that Dean Simon is very involved in the implementation of the remediation plan. In some cases, having the dean involved emphasizes the seriousness of the problem and the high level of concern that the school has over the learner's struggles, as well as their dedication to the learner's education. In other cases, having the dean involved will result in additional anxiety or hesitancy of the learner to disclose necessary personal information. Each circumstance needs to be assessed individually, as well as the character, personality, and approach of the dean and what is best for the learner. Regardless of whether the dean makes final decisions about the learner's progress, there may be a perception that the dean has influence over the learner's successful completion of the program.[7,8] Some learners need a firm remediator, while others need someone to hold their hand. The most skilled and experienced remediators can adapt to the needs of the learner.[9]

With this background, Dean Simon was able to win José's confidence, and José agreed to meet with the dean on a weekly basis to discuss feedback about his performance and review his progress. The dean arranged for José to work with a pediatric chief resident with exemplary communication skills. The specific goal was to improve both his patient interview skills and his verbal patient presentations. These skills did improve over the remaining 4 weeks of José's pediatric clerkship but were still not at a passing level.

After the pediatric clerkship, José started a 6-week inpatient internal medicine clerkship. Once again, the dean was able to arrange for José to be assigned to a team with a senior resident with very strong communication skills. This was not without some challenges, as José was upset that the pediatric residents had reached out to internal medicine residents assigned to work with him to let them know of their concerns. At their weekly meetings, Dean Simon tried to keep José's focus on working to improve communications skills, and not on perceived slights.

During his internal medicine clerkship, José had a negative interaction with an intern who he perceived was treating him unfairly compared to the other student on the team. Both the intern and the supervising senior resident denied that this was the case, and they felt that this accusation was straining the ability of the team to work well together. During their subsequent weekly meeting, Dean Simon asked José to consider the perspective of the other intern. The dean asked José to reflect on how their differences could have been addressed better, before things escalated to the level of a major team conflict.

One other method they employed was to have José take more ownership of his communication problems by asking him to proactively tell attending physicians and supervising residents about his prior communication difficulties and to ask for their assistance in improving his communication skills. He asked them to let him know if they observed any inappropriate behavior with either them or other members of the healthcare team.

> *Editor: Remember, learners who isolate themselves from others are the least successful. Trying to "fly under the radar" until graduation is a path destined for failure. It is most helpful to bring the team in as allies to assist in skill development. Healthcare professionals have "helping" personalities and they will go out of their way to work with a struggling learner if the struggling learner lets them and puts in the effort.*
>
> *Asking for and receiving in-the-moment feedback is ideal. It helps the learner increase their self-awareness and affords them an opportunity to try a different approach in the moment.*[10,11]

By the end of his 6-week internal medicine clerkship, after lots of coaching and input from the senior resident on his team, José was felt to be communicating better. He was doing a better job obtaining complete medical histories from assigned patients, and his verbal patient presentations were better organized and more complete. His reporting skills were assessed to be at a marginal pass level by both the senior resident and the attending physician supervising his performance.

At the dean and José's weekly meeting just before completion of the internal medicine clerkship, José volunteered that he would approach senior resident and attending physician supervisors at the start of each subsequent rotation to share the difficulties he had experienced with communication skills during his prior clerkships. Dean Simon asked José to also allow him to periodically check in with these supervisors to get feedback about his performance. José agreed to this approach. There continued to be issues (none of them major) as José had some difficulty adapting his reporting skills to new methods and formats used on different services. At times, feedback from supervisors suggested José rigidly resisted efforts to help him adjust his reporting skills to the format used on other services.

> *Editor: Here's another example of a learner who struggles with flexibility. Every patient case gets the same presentation or the same note regardless of the circumstances. The learner needs to be taught to consider what the listener*

needs to hear. This is the next step after a student learns how to present a standard history and physical and SOAP note.

DISCIPLINARY ACTION

The promotions committee got involved early, requesting that José meet with them to address a report of unprofessional behavior submitted by the supervising attending physician he worked with on his first clinical (pediatric) clerkship. The professionalism concern was based on the series of incidents observed during that clerkship.

José appeared in person but was poorly prepared for the session. When asked to make an opening statement to the committee, he chose to deny all their concerns. José stated that he felt the entire pediatric care team did not like him and was prejudiced against him. When he was asked to discuss each of the incidents described by the attending physician, he refused to cooperate and stated that all the allegations were false. He felt that he had done nothing wrong and that he had no problem with his data gathering or reporting skills.

The promotions committee felt the concerns raised were real. They recommended that José be placed on academic probation and work with the physician who directs the professional remediation program for the College of Medicine. Until this point, José had not shared with Dean Simon that he had been called to appear before the promotions committee, nor had he discussed with the dean in advance what approach to take in responding to committee concerns. Fortunately, Dean Simon was able to visit with the physician directing the professional remediation program and share his observations from working with José on his communication difficulties for the prior two months.

Editor: It is impressive that the dean dedicated so much time to this learner, but why wasn't the remediation team notified earlier? Even if the dean possessed more experience working with struggling learners, this would have been an opportunity for him to mentor his more junior peers in the remediation process. The remediation team needs to see as many learners as possible to build expertise, work together to build remediation plans, and harness resources.[9,12] Perhaps the remediation team was overwhelmed with other learners and the dean tried to lend a helping hand all around.

Together, Dean Simon and the physician directing the remediation program met with José and explained the consequences of professionalism concerns and probation issues. They impressed upon José that if he were to be placed on probation, he would need to explain these concerns throughout his career. Further consequences could include required monitoring by the licensing board and increased supervision to monitor his interactions with patients and other members of the healthcare team.

With Dean Simon's assistance and coaching, José arranged to have an additional meeting with the promotions committee. At this meeting he read a statement acknowledging his role in the professionalism concerns and communication issues that arose during his pediatric clerkship. He stated that he was working to improve his communication skills and pledged that there would be no further professionalism concerns during his remaining 1+ years in medical school. The promotions committee accepted this response and removed the probation status but stated that any further confirmed incidents could lead to academic probation, or possibly dismissal from school.

Editor: Why was an acknowledgement all that it took for José to be removed from probation? Did anyone retest his competence? Was he performing at the level of an early third-year medical student and had he demonstrated that he could sustain this performance prior to being taken off probation?

Learners often do not realize that it is not only the seriousness of their deficits that lead to probation, but also their response to feedback, the remediation plan, and their willingness to participate in a new learning plan that determine how training programs decide what disciplinary actions to take.[12]

SUCCESSES

A multi-faceted remediation approach was key. Remediation efforts started with requiring José to undergo a mental health evaluation. This was important to assure there wasn't an acute mental health or substance abuse concern. The second step was to identify a physician mentor of the same ethnicity because José was convinced that much of the concern about his performance was based on bias against him due to his Latinx ethnicity. The Latino physician and José met several times, and although they didn't succeed in developing a mentoring relationship, the physician was able to help José understand the need to address his communication issues. The key element to successful remediation was the excellent coaching provided by several senior residents who regularly worked with José to improve his information gathering from patients and his subsequent verbal presentations. Finally, weekly meetings with Dean Simon to monitor José's performance and promptly address any communication issues as they arose were also key to successful remediation.

Fortunately, José was able to avoid any other major professionalism issues. However, he needed continued work on his patient communication and reporting skills throughout the remainder of medical school. Although he improved at informing supervising residents and faculty about his problems in these areas, he needed frequent reminders to accept constructive feedback – without seeing it as personal attacks or assuming criticism was due to his ethnicity (which, with rare exceptions, was the not the case).

José graduated from medical school and became a resident in a program close to his hometown in an area that serves many Latinx patients and most members of the healthcare team are of Latinx ethnicity. Dean Simon has maintained contact with him, and he shares that José is mostly doing well in his intern year, although he has had issues raised about his efficiency in interviewing patients and his ability to adapt his verbal presentation and notes to the format used by different services. There have been no known professionalism concerns to this point in his training.

Editor: In reviewing the literature, there is much written about the lack of academic preparedness of underrepresented minorities (URMs) when they enter medical professional schools. URMs often enter less well prepared than their classmates, having attended weaker high schools with less-skilled teachers and under-resourced science laboratories. URMs often graduate from lower-ranking colleges and universities, and while at college have lower performance due to their poor secondary educational foundations and not knowing about or utilizing academic support services available to them. Within the URM culture, asking for help is often considered a sign of weakness rather than a sign of curiosity and desire to learn. URMs tend to have fewer resources to afford supplementary study materials, practice questions, and board review tools.[13,14,15] While having the innate skills, these learners may suffer from imposter syndrome when they compare themselves to their more-advantaged peers.

URMs also face a lack of racially or ethnically similar mentors who can boost hope during the challenging periods of school, support appropriate levels of confidence, and provide encouragement and a welcoming environment. URMs often must face and combat stereotypes from people who are unlike them. In addition to learning the medical curriculum, they have to learn the new language of medicine and find their way in a culture which is less familiar to them than to peers who grew up in the medical community, having parents and relatives in the medical professions.[3,13,14,15]

Remediation faculty must be aware of the additional challenges placed on URMs who may need and do deserve academic, emotional, financial, and social support. They may need help navigating medicine. They may need assistance balancing home and school obligations, as their families may not understand the demands of training and may have unreasonable expectations of their availability. Keep these factors in mind when choosing tutors, offering additional learning services, connecting peer support or faculty mentors, providing career counseling, and recommending exam preparation tools. Ensure that the remediation team has implicit bias training and don't be afraid to talk about it with the learner. Acknowledge that it exists and will be addressed at the institutional level because diversity is truly an asset. Then move on to what the learner can do to improve their performance.[3] ⊄

REFERENCES

1   Cleland JA, Arnold R, Chesser A. Failing finals is often a surprise for the student but not the teacher. *Med Teach*. 2005;27:504-8.

2   Cleland J, Leggett H, Sandars J, Costa MJ, Patel R, Moffat M. The remediation challenge: theoretical and methodological insights from a systematic review. *Med Educ*.2013;47:242-51.

3   Toretsky C, Mutha S, Coffman J. Breaking barriers for underrepresented minorities in the health professions. Retrieved from Healthforce Center at UCSF website https://healthforce. ucsf.edu/publications/breaking-barriers-underrepresented-minorities-health-professions. 2018 Jul.

4   Holmboe ES, Yepes M, Williams F, Huot SJ. "Feedback and the mini clinical evaluation exercise." *JGIM*. 2004;19(5pt2):558-61.

5   Ellson TJ, David S. Fitness to practice procedures for medical students. *Brit J Hosp Med*. 2015; 76(7) 405-408.

6   Ellson TJ, David S. General Medical Council refusal to grant provisional registration – reasons, prevention and what to do if it happens. *The Brit Stu Doc*. 20017;1(2):36-40.

7   Kalet A, Chou CL, Ellaway RH. To fail is human: remediating remediation in medical education. *Perspect Med Educ*. 2017;6:418-24.

8   Kebaetse MB, Winston K. Physician remediation: accepting and working with complementary conceptualisations. *Med Educ*. 2019;53:210-1.

9   Winston KA, van der Vleuten CP, Scherpbier AJ. The role of the teacher in remediating at risk medical students. *Med Teach*. 2013;34:e732-42.

10   Hewson MG, Little ML. Giving feedback in medical education: verification of recommended techniques. *JGIM*. 1998 Feb;13(2):111-6.

11   Stone D, Heen S. *Thanks for the feedback: The science and art of receiving feedback well (even when it is off base, unfair, poorly delivered, and frankly, you're not in the mood)*. Penguin; 2015.

12   Winston KA, van der Vleuten CP, Scherpbier AJ. Prediction and prevention of failure: An early intervention to assist at-risk medical students. *Med Teach*. 2014 Jan 1;36(1):25-31.

13   Alexander C, Chen E, Grumbach K. How leaky is the health career pipeline? Minority student achievement in college gateway courses. *Acad Med*. 2009;84(6):797-802.

14   Barr DA, Matsui J, Wanat SF, Gonzalez ME. Chemistry courses as the turning point for premedical students. *Adv Health Sci Educ Theory Pract*. 2010;15(1):45-54.

15   Barr DA, Gonzalez ME, Wanat SF. The leaky pipeline: Factors associated with early decline in interest in premedical studies among underrepresented minority undergraduate students. *Acad Med*. 2008;83(5):503-511.

CASE 18

Professionalism

LEARNER AT TIME OF IDENTIFICATION FOR REMEDIATION

Emily, a fourth post-graduate year resident in urology

REASON FOR REMEDIATION

Emily was referred to her institution's centralized coaching and remediation program by her program director for concerns related to professionalism. There had been several nursing complaints about Emily's short temper and angry outbursts, observed particularly when she was under stress. She frequently snapped at nurses when on call saying things like, "Why are you torturing me?" or, "Why can't you just do your job?" She once stormed out of the emergency department mid-procedure when a nurse disrupted her sterile field. Her peers complained that she was "not a team player" and "has no filter." Specifically, she frequently objected to being overworked and "has a temper tantrum every time she is called in [while on home call]." She rarely helped out when there were cases that required staying late.

REMEDIATION APPROACH

Dr. Jules worked with Emily as her primary coach. They met 15 times (60-90 minutes each) over a period of 6 months, one-on-one, in person, in Dr. Jules' office.

Meeting 1 – Objectives: Build rapport, gain understanding of learner perspective on the issues that led to referral, gauge insight and willingness/ability to reflect, explore for the presence of underlying issues related to mental well-being

Emily was open and reflective and demonstrated some insight into the behaviors that had led to the referral. She understood the reason for the referral. By self-report, the other aspects of Emily's clinical performance in residency were average/slightly above average (technical skill, medical knowledge, clinical reasoning). She had never been on remediation and did well in medical school. Emily expressed that she didn't feel supported by her program. She didn't have a mentor and didn't feel that the program director "has her back." She reported that she has good local support, exercises regularly, does not abuse substances, and on days off engages in hobbies that make her feel renewed. She denied any history of mental illness and has never seen a therapist.

Emily struggles with subjective anxiety on call and tends to catastrophize. She worries about things that might happen – bad outcomes, getting called back into the hospital, being tired the next day. She perseverates about phone calls she has already received. She frequently experiences frustration with the nursing staff and makes many statements to the effect of "they should know how to put in this urinary catheter," "they should have tried harder before they called me," and "they are just trying to torture me because they know I'm on call."

Dr. Jules gave her the following instruments to fill out prior to meeting 2: GAD-7, PHQ-9, Gottman's flooding self-test, and the MBI.

Editor: GAD stands for generalized anxiety disorder, PHQ for personalized health questionnaire, and MBI for Maslach burnout inventory. The first screening instrument assesses for anxiety, the second for depression, Gottman's test for emotional flooding, and the MBI for symptoms of burnout. It is a very fine line to walk between helping a struggling learner and being their clinician, and the boundaries here are beginning to blur. While the data can be extremely helpful for both the remediator (if trained to use these tools) and the learner, these assessments are best done by an independent clinician who can then share the results. It is important for faculty to demonstrate clear boundaries with learners, as we serve as role models for many struggling learners who themselves are challenged with boundary issues.[1]

Meeting 2 – Objectives: Review instruments, introduce the circle of concern/circle of influence, basics of mindful communication, review of triggers

The PHQ-9 score was not suggestive of a depressive disorder. The GAD-7 revealed mild anxiety. Emily's flooding score was quite elevated, suggesting that she is prone to feeling flooded during conflict. Her MBI was notable for moderate emotional exhaustion, high depersonalization, and high personal accomplishment. Dr. Jules and Emily reviewed these briefly and laid out plans to discuss the results in more detail in subsequent meetings.

Together they reviewed Stephen Covey's circle of influence/circle of concern. Dr. Jules pointed out that Emily was spending a lot of time in her circle of concern, worrying about things that she cannot control. They brainstormed strategies to shift Emily's focus to the circle of influence while on call. Dr. Jules provided a handout reinforcing the concept of problem-focused coping strategies for issues within the circle of influence, and emotion-focused coping strategies for issues within the circle of concern.

> *Editor: Picture one circle drawn inside another. Stephen Covey's circle of influence exists embedded within the circle of concern. An individual's circle of influence includes the things that cause concern that they can do something about. Things that live outside of the circle of influence but within the circle of concern are things that create concern, but one has no control over.[2] For instance, Emily may worry about how many more phone calls will come in before the night is over. This is outside of her control, but within her circle of concern. She may be embarrassed by others' reactions to her behaviors and that she is perceived as having temper tantrums. That lives within her circle of influence and within her circle of concern.*

Dr. Jules and Emily discussed that, when interacting with others, individuals are influenced both by their own history and interpersonal characteristics and the other's history and interpersonal characteristics. They reviewed the importance of nonverbal communication and Emily's communication style, specifically how she comes across when triggered. They discovered that Emily tends to roll her eyes, raise her voice, "huff and puff," and even slam doors when she is triggered. She was aware of the facial expressions and changes in the quality of her voice that occur when she is upset.

Reflecting on her triggers, Emily admitted that she often believes there is only one right way to do something. She gets frustrated when others are doing things that she perceives as "wrong," or when others are what she perceives as "incompetent." Emily is triggered when she feels that others are not thoughtful of her time, when people "don't do their job," and when others tell her what to do. She is also triggered by not feeling heard or seen; specifically, it bothers her when others don't seem to appreciate how hard she is working. Her threshold for being triggered is lowered significantly by lack of sleep and the anxiety of being on call. She described the following scenario: "I was asked to stay late to do a complex case in the operating room. I immediately reacted and stormed out of the room. No one gets that I was here late last night. I want to make my own decisions. I gave the case to one of the second-year residents. I know this makes me a selfish person. I feel bad about it."

Dr. Jules gave her the following homework assignment: Consider the spoken and unspoken values or rules that were clear in your family of origin. What patterns or traditions in your family of origin helped you become successful? What patterns or traditions set you up for your present difficulties or other problems? Was high achievement valued in your family? How were conflicts settled in your family?

Meeting 3 – Objectives: Understand the family system, explore origins of triggers

Examining their family system helps learners to recognize patterns within that system. Recognition of these patterns can help avoid repeating or transmitting them in the future. Dr. Jules and Emily reviewed the homework assignment and discussed that one's triggers, or maps, are the result of rules that were learned early in life. These are often activated when one perceives that people have done things that they shouldn't have. Each individual has a unique map, and when they apply their rules to other people, this may trigger a strong emotional response.

Emily grew up in a highly competitive household where achievement was paramount and approval was rarely expressed. Her father is a highly accomplished surgeon whose identity is defined by his work. He is known at work for his explosive temper, and he is beloved by all his patients. Emily is the middle child; two of her siblings are physicians. In her household, it was an important unspoken value that emotions are a sign of weakness.

Anger was the only emotion that was regularly expressed. Conflicts were handled in a very top-down manner, and there was always a clear winner and loser – with no middle ground. Emily remembers getting attention by acting out and being rebellious. She rarely felt heard or seen by her parents. She described growing up thinking that competence is defined by an aggressive communication style and apologies are a sign of weakness. She developed a black-and-white style of thinking and has always struggled with the idea of compromise. Emily eventually began to see that her lifelong struggle to be heard had led to her being triggered at work when others don't recognize how hard she is working.

> *Editor: While her father's explosive temper may have been tolerated in the medical environment back when he trained and practiced, that is no longer the case. It might benefit Emily to include in the conversation how expectations around physician behavior have evolved along with our understand of how physician behavior impacts patient outcomes.*

Meeting 4 – Objectives: Review the concept of flooding and the importance of mindfulness in the moment, introduce concept of means-end thinking, fundamental attribution error, and assuming positive intent

Emily's score on Gottman's flooding self-test was high. This was commensurate with her reflections on how she feels and behaves when triggered and in line with the observations leading to her referral. The key to mitigating a high flooding score is promoting awareness in the moment. With a better understanding of (a) what her triggers are, (b) how she feels when triggered, and (c) how she often reacts when triggered, they were able to move to the concept of mindfulness in the moment. Dr. Jules introduced the STOP exercise (S: pause for a moment; T: take a breath to calm; O: observe what I'm feeling, identify my goals and my choices; P: proceed with awareness). They discussed the importance of moving from reacting to responding. They role-played scenarios based on situations that triggered Emily in the workplace.

Next, Emily and Dr. Jules discussed the concept of means-end thinking, which is the ability to orient oneself and conceptualize the means of moving toward a goal. In situations in which she is triggered, Dr. Jules suggested that Emily ask herself what she wants out of the interaction or the other person. They explored the importance of, whenever possible, visualizing herself aligned with the other person as though they are on the same side looking at a problem together. Yelling at a nurse is unlikely to accomplish anything other than making the nurse behave passive-aggressively. They discussed the importance of setting a goal that is realistic and within Emily's circle of influence. They role-played additional scenarios and practiced those skills.

Dr. Jules and Emily also reviewed the concept of fundamental attribution error, which is one's bias toward assigning motivation to why other people do what they do. When Emily was under stress, she tended to assume that nurses were calling her because they were incompetent or lazy. Emily and Dr. Jules discussed that jumping to this conclusion is fundamentally a cognitive error, based on no data. If Emily were to assume positive intent, e.g., that people are just trying to do their jobs, she would experience greater satisfaction and interpersonal effectiveness.

Emily's homework was to explore some of the resources Dr. Jules provided on mindfulness and meditation and to keep track of interpersonal interactions that both went well and not so well.

Meeting 5 – Objectives: Review burnout and its components, strategies for mitigating the high depersonalization score

Emily's high depersonalization score seemed to be a natural outgrowth of her being triggered by things that she cannot control (difficult patients, difficult interactions with support staff, calls on an on-call night). Dr. Jules reviewed that Emily will be put in positions during her training in which she is asked to do things she feels she shouldn't have to do, and it's natural to make the patient or the nurse a part of this narrative. The trick here is to be aware and understand where this feeling comes from. Her burnout score will likely be lowered when she gets past these "shoulds" and shifts energy from the circle of concern to the circle of influence.

Emily shared her experience thus far with the practice of mindfulness, which had begun as an exploration of the Headspace app on her phone. They reviewed some examples of interpersonal interactions in which she employed the STOP exercise when she felt herself being triggered. In one incident, Emily was performing a procedure which was being delayed because the X-ray technician was having trouble completing the X-ray. Frustrated and flustered, Emily raised her voice and became aggressive with the technician, causing the technician to move even more slowly. Emily recognized that her communication style did not bring about her desired result, but she was stuck on her preconceived notion that being "overly nice" was a sign of weakness. Dr. Jules reviewed the connection of this belief to Emily's family of origin and used the incident as an opportunity to role-play scenarios in which she tried a different approach with the technician, ultimately landing a communication style that was more assertive than aggressive.

Emily's homework was to continue keeping track of interpersonal interactions that went both well and not so well.

Meetings 6-15

With the insights and skills gained in their earlier meetings, Emily began to make significant progress. Dr. Jules explored Emily's triggers with her in more detail. They spent a lot of time on her reactions in situations in which she felt she was being told what to do and in which she had little control. She grew to recognize that her response in these situations was to push back, or even refuse to do the work. This had led to the development of a reputation among her peers as someone who tries to get out of work, which was distressing to Emily, who values a good work ethic and very much wants to be seen as a hard worker. She remembered pushing boundaries as a young child and into adolescence. "I never wanted to do what other people told me to do. I wanted to make my own decisions. I got attention by being rebellious." Once she became aware of her tendency to do this and understood that her pushback and refusals were not in fact about being lazy but rather about being triggered by feeling unheard or out of control, she was able to reliably pause in the moment and respond in a more effective way. Emily began to stay later at work, sign out less cases to her peers, and take on more complex cases. She found this rewarding and received a lot of positive feedback from her attending physicians.

In one meeting, Emily reflected on an interaction with a nurse in the emergency department in which a nurse disposed of some of Emily's equipment after she had inadvertently left it sitting in an unoccupied room. Emily remembered that she and Dr. Jules had discussed the practice of assuming positive intent and concluded that the nurse was simply trying to do her job and maintain a safe workplace. Emily confronted the nurse but, instead of yelling, she apologized for leaving the equipment out in the open and unattended in the room. This was very uncomfortable for Emily, given her longstanding belief that apologies are a sign of weakness. She reported being surprised that the nurse "immediately backed down," and that she "felt really good about the whole thing." In the end, she had made a conscious decision to enter into a collaborative relationship with the nurse.

Over time, Emily reported greater satisfaction in her work. She felt happier and more present both at home and at work. She was consistently able to pause in the moment when triggered and choose her response. As she began staying later and taking on extra and more complex cases, she was relieved to note that this felt good. Emily and Dr. Jules spent a few sessions talking about her reputation – which she had initially claimed not to care about but, as she discovered, was very important to her. She developed an increased awareness that she had developed a reputation as someone who was not a team player and tried to get out of work. She began to develop "money in the bank," becoming intentional about being more positive and willing to help others at work. She found that this led to greater satisfaction – even when she put in longer hours.

As her situation improved, Emily began meeting with Dr. Jules monthly instead of weekly, and now she checks in on an as-needed basis. Her program director and chair have been pleased with her performance.

DISCIPLINARY ACTION

None. Referral to her institution's program is a pre-disciplinary process.

SUCCESSES

Helping Emily to raise awareness around her triggers, the origins of her triggers, and her reactions when triggered was a very empowering experience for her. It ultimately helped her to learn to respond rather than react in the moment in a way that made her more interpersonally effective.

The program was successful. Emily is now subjectively much happier at work and is off the radar of her program director.

HINDSIGHT REFLECTIONS FROM THE REMEDIATING FACULTY

Emily would have benefitted from working with a therapist who specializes in family systems. We suggested this on many occasions and, in retrospect, might have pushed harder for it to happen.

Editor: Dr. Jules showed remarkable skills in devising a thoughtful, organized, intentional series of meetings with progress agendas. She was able to make acute observations in the learner, adapt her responses accordingly, respond authentically, and provide reliable support and appropriate feedback and encouragement. Not all remediators will have the same level of psychological understanding or ability, but that doesn't mean you can't be successful in helping struggling learners. This case gives an amazing framework that can serve as a model for less-experienced remediators to adopt and adapt based on their own style and the learner in front of them. It is a phenomenal outline that gets to the deepest levels of reflections to allow a struggling learner to accept feedback, understand the consequences of their behavior, and begin to change their behavior for the better. 💬

REFERENCES

1   Paice E, Heard S, Moss F. How important are role models in making good doctors? *BMJ.* 2002 Sep 28;325(7366):707-10.

2   Covey S. *The 7 Habits of Highly Effective People.* Habit 2. New York, Simon and Schuster; 1989.

CASE 19

Clinical Reasoning

LEARNER AT TIME OF IDENTIFICATION FOR REMEDIATION

Doug, an end-of-the-year, first post-graduate year resident in family medicine

REASON FOR REMEDIATION

Doug was referred to his institution's centralized coaching and remediation program because of concerns related to his performance on the inpatient general medicine service. He struggled with oral patient presentations and progress notes. Specifically, information was out of order, key information was missing, and his problem list was not ordered appropriately in terms of severity of problem. His differential diagnoses were narrow and often missed important items. He exhibited premature closure and required close supervision and assistance to create appropriate management plans for his patients. Doug's performance was acceptable in clinic as long as the pace was slow and patients were straightforward. There was concern about him transitioning to the role of a supervising resident the following month. He had been told that he needed to improve his medical knowledge and develop an effective reading plan.

When the institution's assessment team reviewed Doug's performance in medical school, they noted that he had performed in the third quartile of his class. His subject exam scores were slightly below average, with no test failures. Positive comments from the core clerkships highlighted his excellent interpersonal skills, humility, and strong work ethic. One evaluator acknowledged that his presentations "improved over the course of the rotation." His United States Medical Licensing Examination (USMLE) Step I and II scores were in the 230s (50th and 47th percentile respectively) with no test failures.

> *Editor: Struggling learners are disproportionately referred for remediation for medical knowledge deficits, when in fact the deficit usually lies in other categories. In this case, with near-average exam scores, Doug should have had enough knowledge to perform adequately.[1] Clearly, medical knowledge was not the main problem, and the all-too-often generic recommended remediation strategy of "reading more" was not going to solve his problem.[2] Given that he has sufficient knowledge, Doug needs to learn how to apply it to the patient in front of him. This is not something that can be learned from a book alone.*

REMEDIATION APPROACH

The institution's clinical reasoning coaching program involves three phases:

Phase 1 – Learners are referred to a centralized coaching and remediation program, either by their program director or by self-referral. A remediation specialist performs a standardized assessment using a biopsychosocial approach that consists of reviewing available evaluative data and performance in prior programs and courses, followed by a face-to-face interview with the learner. A primary clinical performance deficit is identified using the following categorization: medical knowledge, clinical reasoning, organization/efficiency, professionalism, communication, and operative skill. For those with a primary clinical reasoning deficit, the learner moves to Phase 2.

Editor: Over 30% of struggling learners bring something personal into the learning environment that impacts their ability to perform: mental health disorders, physical illness, life stress that doesn't rise to the level of a mental health diagnosis (e.g., a newborn, an ill parent, a divorce), burnout, learning disorders.[3,4,5] *The editor categorizes these external factors into a bucket labeled well-being, which could be added to the list above. In this case, it would be important to make sure Doug isn't suffering from anything such as narcolepsy or medication side effects that could affect his cognitive horsepower. The editor once had a learner referred for poor clinical decisions in the operating room that was ultimately caused by a previously undiagnosed congenital vision problem. Think outside the box, but don't get lost there.*

When taking into consideration the information provided by the undergraduate medical record, the concerns noted by Doug's evaluators were most consistent with a clinical reasoning deficit. A significant medical knowledge deficit can masquerade as a clinical reasoning deficit. It is true that one cannot apply knowledge that one does not possess. However, in this case, Doug seemed to struggle even in situations where his knowledge of the disease process was sufficient.

Phase 2 – In this program, learners with a primary clinical reasoning deficit are referred to a clinical reasoning coach to initiate a clinical reasoning remediation program. The program begins with weekly one-on-one coaching sessions that include a review of key concepts in clinical reasoning, including cognitive biases with de-biasing strategies and dual process reasoning. Using handouts and online videos, the coach employs case-based reasoning exercises to target the specific clinical reasoning deficit along the following pathway (see **Figure 19.1**): hypothesis generation, data collection, problem representation, refinement of hypotheses, development of a working diagnosis (script selection), and management. Though the simplicity and linear nature of this pathway is not completely realistic, this process allows the coach to identify specific deficits amenable to targeted intervention. Doug was asked to methodically work through cases in this stepwise fashion, with repeated prompting from the coach to think aloud.

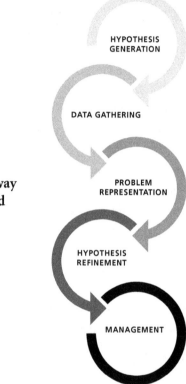

FIGURE 19.1

Linear clinical reasoning pathway used for targeted remediation

Doug's coach presented him with an evidence-based framework for diagnostic and management reasoning, similar to that depicted in the figure above. The coach applied this process as they worked their way through multiple clinical cases. For the most part, Doug had a solid clinical knowledge base but struggled with knowledge organization to the point where it was difficult to apply it efficiently. The coach thus focused on imparting a systematic process that Doug could apply to every patient, over time becoming more natural and efficient. The coach determined that the primary breakdown in the clinical reasoning pathway was hypothesis generation, prior to the patient encounter.

To address this, Doug was encouraged to use System-2 based schema in generating an early, broad differential diagnosis. This was in addition to the System-1 based pattern recognition that he already possessed.

Editor: As a reminder, System 1 refers to implicit, automatic, pattern recognition decision making or nonanalytical reasoning. System 2 refers to explicit, controlled, rational, effortful, relatively slow analytical reasoning.[6]

Pre-test Probability

Consider the probability of suspected diseases based on their prevalence, specific to a given patient. Common diseases are common.

Anatomical

What lives there? Consider the organs and surrounding structures in a given location and what can go wrong with each.

Pathophysiology

Consider the physiological processes of disease leading to the chief complaint.

Systems

Consider various organ systems and disease processes in each.

Worst-Case Scenario

Consider conditions that can lead to mortality or significant morbidity specific to a given patient. These are cannot-miss diagnoses.

In Phase 2, Doug met with his coach weekly (60 minutes each) for 1 month, one-on-one. The coach spent 8 hours preparing for the coaching sessions.

Phase 3 – Lessons learned through work with the clinical reasoning coach are then fed forward to faculty and/or peer evaluators for use during subsequent direct observation in the clinical learning environment. Building on data from the global and targeted assessment of the learner, the coach gathers real-time feedback from these evaluators and, when necessary, provides education regarding the assessment and coaching of clinical reasoning in the clinical learning environment.

> *Editor: In speaking with those involved with hundreds of programs, feeding information forward to subsequent evaluators seems to be the most controversial subtopic within remediation. The Rosenthal or Pygmalion effect is a true phenomenon in which high expectations can lead to improved performance and low expectations can lead to lower performance.[7] However, it is also true that remediation does not occur quickly. It spans several courses, rotations, and sometimes academic years.[8,9,10] It becomes necessary to feed*

information forward to propagate the remediation plan, ensure that the learners are getting timely feedback, and give the learners opportunities to practice in the areas in which they are deficient.[11,12,13,14,15,16] If each attending approaches a struggling learner blindly, the attending physician will spend all of their short time together trying to identify the problem rather than helping to remediate it.[17] And each attending physician will not have the benefit of input from teachers who have more experience and expertise working with struggling learners.[18] Our ultimate goal is to make sure that our learners are successful and competent when they graduate.

This institution's program has developed an interdepartmental clinical reasoning coaching committee in an effort to train members in a standardized approach to the diagnosis and coaching of clinical reasoning deficits among graduate medical learners and to develop durable materials that a variety of academic departments at the institution can use for coaching. They had identified two faculty members from Doug's department who were interested in remediation and had received some faculty development around clinical reasoning coaching. The clinical reasoning coach worked with these faculty members to transition the coaching program to the department level in Phase 3.

Doug was initially uncomfortable soliciting feedback on his performance and feeding information forward to his evaluators; however, he gave permission for his coach to do so. Over time he became more comfortable with this skill and gained proficiency in it. Doug was given a worksheet to practice with every patient. Using the previously described frameworks, he was encouraged to take five minutes to create a broad differential diagnosis before seeing the patient based simply upon the chief complaint.

Editor: Giving Doug time to prepare prior to a patient encounter increases his ability to create broad differential diagnoses. It also allows him to ask more effective questions and perform more pertinent physical exam maneuvers during the patient encounter while anticipating a possible diagnostic work-up. This will allow him to work on efficiency during the entire encounter.

The departmental clinical competency committee met at months 3 and 6 following the initial referral and concluded that Doug's performance had improved significantly. At month 6 the formal coaching program ended. The clinical reasoning coach has stayed in touch with Doug, who reports that he is still using the frameworks and tools learned in Phase 2.

> *Editor: Had Doug learned these skills as a third-year medical student, can you imagine how much more he would have learned from each patient encounter during his clinical clerkships and acting-internship? Are we teaching students clinical reasoning skills in a way that is effective? At your institution, is there a better way of identifying those that need additional teaching before they are handed the reins of more independent decision making, as in this case? It is hard to imagine that no one knew this was a problem previously. Had Doug's problem been identified sooner, the second-year class would not be short a member and there would have been less disruption to the workforce.*
>
> *We still receive reports of faculty questioning their ability to detect those who need remediation and who don't meet the minimal standards, and being unsure of the process of identifying struggling learners. Faculty development can be provided to support them in the early identification of struggling learners, diagnosis of the learner's deficits, effective early interventions, and when and where it is appropriate to refer a struggling learner.[19,20]*

DISCIPLINARY ACTION

None. Referral to the institution's program is a pre-disciplinary process.

SUCCESSES

Doug was referred several months after his struggles were noted by his program, at a critical transition point (moving from intern to supervising resident). Although Doug's struggles were recognized by his program as early as October of his intern year, as evidenced by confidential comments to the program director, there was little in the written evaluations to suggest that he lagged behind his peers. Experience shows that there is often a delay in recognition, or willingness to admit recognition, of struggling learners. There are many potential barriers: remediation is time-consuming, perceived stigma to the learner, lack of comfort or skills with remediation, logistic challenges, and fear of retribution. Because remediation – particularly clinical reasoning remediation – takes time, early recognition of struggle is critical.

In Doug's case, the delay occurred because his program was worried that he might have felt stigmatized by the referral for coaching and that this may have hindered his progress. In hindsight, it was clear that Doug was quite aware that he was struggling and already stigmatized, long prior to referral. The program had to make some changes to his schedule as part of the transition from intern to resident, given that he was not yet ready to lead a team on the inpatient service at the time of initial referral. Had the referral for coaching occurred 3-6 months earlier, this likely could have been avoided.

Editor: What can be done at your institution to destigmatize remediation? [21,22,23] *At one institution the longstanding dean openly speaks about having to repeat his first year of medical school. Everyone struggles at one time or another during training. Seeking help is normal. When was the last time you called a consult? Asked a colleague a question, even if it was about your parent's illness and not a patient? Called someone from another discipline with a question? How many times this week? This needs to be normalized as part of the culture of learning in medicine. Medicine is a team sport.*

HINDSIGHT REFLECTIONS FROM THE REMEDIATING FACULTY

Our program is always working to streamline communication between coaches and departmental evaluators. In this case there were some hiccups in the transition from Phase 2 to Phase 3 that could have been avoided had we sat down for an hour to make the transition more formal. We have now incorporated this into the protocol and anticipate that things will move more smoothly going forward.

REFERENCES

1   Wiese JG. "Strong as Our Weakest Link." Presentation, Tulane University Health Sciences Center. 2006.

2   Audetat Voirol MC, Laurin S, Dory V. Remediation for struggling learners: putting an end to "more of the same." *Med Educ.* 2013;47(3):230-1.

3   Guerrasio J, Garrity MJ, Aagaard EM. Learner deficits and academic outcomes of medical students, residents, fellows, and attending physicians referred to a remediation program, 2006-2012. *Acad Med.* 2014 Feb 1;89(2):352-8.

4   Yellin PB. Learning differences and medical education. In: Kalet A, Chou CL, editors. *Remediation in Medical Education: A mid-course correction.* Heidelberg, Berlin, New York: Springer;2014.

5   Yates J. Development of a "toolkit" to identify medical students at risk of failure to thrive on the course: an exploratory retrospective case study. *BMC Med Educ.* 2011;11:95.

6   Kahneman D. A perspective on judgment and choice: mapping bounded rationality. *Am Psychol.* 2003; 58(9):697-720.

7   Boser U, Wilhelm M, Hanna R. The power of the Pygmalion effect: teachers' expectations strongly predict college completion. *Center for American Progress.* 2014 Oct 6.

8   Warburton KM, Goren E, Dine CJ. Comprehensive assessment of struggling learners referred to a graduate medical education remediation program. *JGME.* 2017 Dec;9(6):763-7.

9   Zbieranowski I, Takahashi SG, Verma S, Spadafora SM. Remediation of residents in difficulty: a retrospective 10-year review of the experience of a postgraduate board of examiners. *Acad Med.* 2013 Jan 1;88(1):111-6.

10   Guerrasio J, Garrity MJ, Aagaard EM. Learner deficits and academic outcomes of medical students, residents, fellows, and attending physicians referred to a remediation program, 2006-2012. *Acad Med.* 2014 Feb 1;89(2):352-8.

11   Gold WL, McArdle P, Federman DD. Should medical school faculty see assessments of students made by previous teachers? *Acad Med.* 2002;77:1096-100.

12   Price JA. Sharing student background information with faculty: does it make a difference? Dissertation, Harvard University; 2012.

13   Cleary L. "Forward feeding" about students' progress: the case for longitudinal, progressive, and shared assessment of medical students. *Acad Med.* 2008;83:800.

14   Cohen GS, Blumberg P. Investigating whether teachers should be given assessments of students made by previous teachers. *Acad Med.* 1991;66:288-9.

15   Pangaro L. "Forward feeding" about students' progress: more information will enable better policy. *Acad Med.* 2008;83:802-3.

16   Warm EJ, Englander R, Pereira A, Barach P. Improving learner handovers in medical education. *Acad Med.* 2017;92:927-31.

17   Guerrasio J, Brooks E, Rumack CM, Christensen A, Aagaard EM. Association of characteristics, deficits, and outcomes of residents placed on probation at one institution, 2002-2012. *Acad Med.* 2016 Mar 1;91(3):382-7.

18   Winston KA, van der Vleuten CP, Scherpbier AJ. The role of the teacher in remediating at risk medical students. *Med Teach.* 2013; 34:e732-42.

19   Cleland JA, Knight L, Rees C, Tracey S, Bond CB. "Is it me or is it them?" Factors influencing assessors' failure to report underperformance in medical students. *Med Educ.* 2008;42:800-9.

20   Dudek NL, Marks MB, Regehr G. Failure to fail: the perspectives of clinical supervisors. *Acad Med.* 2005 Oct 1;80(10):S84-7.

21   Cutrer WB, Miller B, Pusic MV, et al. Fostering the development of master adaptive learners: a conceptual model to guide skill acquisition in medical education. *Acad Med.* 2017;92:70-5.

22   Bennion LD, Durning SJ, LaRochelle J, et al. Untying the Gordian knot: remediation problems in medical schools that need remediation. *BMC Med Educ.* 2018;18:120.

23   Chou CL, Kalet A, Costa MJ, et al. Guidelines: the dos, don'ts and don't knows of remediation in medical education. *Perspect Med Educ.* 2019;8:322-338.

CASE 20

Clinical Reasoning

LEARNER AT TIME OF IDENTIFICATION FOR REMEDIATION

Allison, a first post-graduate year in pediatrics

REASON FOR REMEDIATION

Allison was referred to her institution's centralized coaching and remediation program for concerns related to communication. Her verbal handovers were noted to be ineffective because they often omitted important details, and her written signouts/handovers did not reflect a good understanding of "the big picture" with her patients. Consulting teams had complained that she didn't seem to know her patients and couldn't communicate "the question" when calling a consult. The parents of one of her patients had relayed to her supervising physician that Allison was unable to convey clearly what was going on with their child. Allison's medical knowledge (as assessed by prior standardized test scores) and command of factual knowledge in conferences were average. She was otherwise thriving in residency and denied any concerns related to mental well-being.

Editor: Some people are right-hand dominant, while others tend to rely on their left hand more. Despite innate handedness, each individual is clearly capable of using both hands. The same is true for how people view situations. Some people see the big picture more easily (the forest) and others see the details (trees) first. Those who see the forest before the trees tend to be better at prioritizing tasks but may miss small details. They make the diagnosis and miss the details in the plan. Those who see the trees first believe that everything is important and needs to be done perfectly and miss the larger picture. They may address every abnormal lab value yet miss the overarching diagnoses. No matter which an individual prefers, they can be taught to double check that they have also viewed the situation from the other perspective.

REMEDIATION APPROACH

Clinical reasoning deficits can be initially miscategorized as problems with communication. In this case, Allison struggled with multiple forms of communication lacking clear, concise information: handoffs, calling consults, and conveying information to patients and their family members. She otherwise had no trouble communicating with other people outside of the clinical environment. Allison also struggled with problem representation. Problem representation refers to the organization of pertinent data into a summary statement, formed through conversion of specific features of the patient's presentation into semantic qualifiers. Formation of an accurate and concise problem representation stimulates the generation of a prioritized list of hypotheses or possible diagnoses through comparison with their stored illness scripts. This "one-liner" then becomes the basis of each of the following: the oral presentation's "assessment," the handoff's updated summary statement, and the consult in the form of an introduction to the patient's current condition and "the question." This skill may develop naturally for some learners, while for others, explicit training is required.

Allison was referred to her institution's clinical reasoning coaching program and assigned a clinical reasoning coach. The first session began with a review of fundamental clinical reasoning concepts and terminology including introduction to the clinical reasoning pathway, a linear stepwise progression of diagnostic and management reasoning processes (hypothesis generation, data collection, problem representation, refinement of hypotheses, development of a working diagnosis (script selection), and management). She was then asked to methodically work through cases in this stepwise fashion, with repeated prompting from her coach to think aloud. This process allowed the coach to identify specific deficits amenable to targeted intervention. In this case, Allison repeatedly struggled to construct an accurate and concise problem representation, confirming the initial assumption. Over a series of three additional 1-hour sessions, the coach introduced the following exercises:

Highlighter – In the highlighter exercise, the learner identifies key clinical features in a written H&P based on possible diagnoses. The clinical reasoning coach asked Allison to bring in a recent admission note and a highlighter. The coach then watched her highlight the key features in the note and provided feedback on her selections. Because accurate and concise problem representations require identification and selection of key data, both pertinent positives and negatives, this exercise is usually effective.

> *Editor: If the learner uses two different color highlighters, they can highlight the evidence for and against their top diagnosis on their differential with two different colors. Or, multiple copies of the same H&P can be made, with each sheet representing a possible diagnosis on their differential. Then the learner can highlight the evidence for and against each of the diagnoses on their differential. If green is for and red is against, the diagnosis corresponding to the copy with the most green highlighting is most likely the front-running diagnosis.*[1]

Priming for co-selection – In this exercise, the learner outlines a differential diagnosis based on the chief complaint alone, then proposes three diagnoses, followed by five questions and five exam findings in an effort to promote hypothesis-driven reasoning. This exercise ensures that data gathering is streamlined. The collected data should then be organized into a problem representation.

Articulated problem representation – The learner is asked to generate a one-line summary of the patient after being presented with a case by the coach. Allison's coach asked her to bring her patient list to meetings, and he selected patients at random from the list for this exercise. The coach critiqued Allison's suggestions by simplifying each problem representation into 3 core components: (1) demographics and risk factors, (2) the temporal pattern of the illness, and (3) key symptoms and signs.

Reverse presentation – This exercise involves having the learner begin the presentation with the assessment to prime for feedback on selection and organization of subjective and objective data.

At the completion of 4 one-hour sessions, Allison was encouraged to continue to practice the skill of developing an effective problem representation under direct observation from her supervising attendings and residents. It was suggested that she feed forward to her supervisors that she was working on this skill and would like feedback and modeling with time for reflection in real time. This worked well for a handful of carefully selected residents and attending physicians over the next month. Gradually, Allison's mastery of these skills grew, and her evaluations reflected that she no longer struggled with handoffs of care or calling consults. There were no additional complaints from patients or family members about how she communicated important information. There have been no concerns about her performance since. Allison is now a third-year resident and obtained a job in private practice following graduation.

DISCIPLINARY ACTION

None. Referral to this program is a pre-disciplinary process.

SUCCESSES

Allison was fully engaged in the process of coaching and was comfortable feeding forward information about the skills she was working on and asking for feedback once coaching was transitioned from the coach's office to the clinical learning environment. This can be very challenging for some learners, and the coaching progress may be halted at this step. When that happens, a fifth coaching session is often devoted to the topic of empowering the learner to seek out feedback and practice actuating that feedback. In this case, role-plays and development of scripts can be effective, followed by frequent check-ins with the learner as they gain comfort applying these skills in the clinical learning environment.

HINDSIGHT REFLECTIONS FROM THE REMEDIATING FACULTY

Learning to formulate an effective problem representation is such a critical area of competence that we would like to be more deliberate about teaching it in our training programs. This skill can be honed in morning report or on rounds by having trainees summarize complex cases in a "one-liner" under direct observation by their peers and faculty facilitators. ⏏

REFERENCES

1   Blankenburg R. Long M. Rosenbluth G. Marisco N. Johnstone N. Dunagan M. Pantaleoni J. Augustine E. Stuart E. "Revisiting how we think: Innovative ideas for promoting and assessing clinical reasoning." *PAS.* May 2011.

CASE 21

Medical Knowledge and Clinical Reasoning

LEARNER AT TIME OF IDENTIFICATION FOR REMEDIATION

Hope, a first post-graduate year resident in internal medicine

REASON FOR REMEDIATION

Hope started her first post-graduate (PGY-1) year in the internal medicine residency program facing challenges that affect the majority of interns: familiarizing herself with a new healthcare system, adjusting to managing a much larger patient load than that of a medical student, and providing clinical assessments about patient management on rounds with much less available time for making clinical decisions.

Many interns gradually transition from the "reporter/interpreter" stage to the "interpreter/manager" stage several months into the PGY-1 year. In Hope's case, however, six months into her PGY-1 year, attendings noted that she remained at the level of a reporter. For example, when rounding with her team on a patient experiencing acute hypotension and a newly low hemoglobin, she struggled to independently formulate a differential diagnosis and management plan for her patient at the time of the clinical event and deferred the entirety of clinical decisions to her supervisors while dutifully placing the orders they had suggested. She was noted to be visibly anxious when she was required to come up with a differential diagnosis and management plan under time pressure. In the outpatient setting, her history-taking was not always hypothesis-driven. For example, in evaluating a patient who endorsed intermittent chest pain in clinic, she missed asking the patient about certain historical details to help discern between angina or more benign causes, and her supervisor had to repeat the history to correctly triage the patient's symptom.

Finally, Hope struggled with time management even during the latter half of her PGY-1 year. She would often miss presenting key items of history, physical exam, or labs during rounds that were pertinent to clinical decision-making for her patients. For example, ineffective time management and a lack of hypothesis-driven pre-rounding caused her to miss reviewing the electrocardiogram for a patient with acute coronary syndrome and the creatinine value for a patient with acute kidney injury.

These performance concerns, noted during the latter half of her intern year, indicated that Hope may struggle during the transition from a PGY-1 to a PGY-2, when she would assume the role of a senior resident who would be required to make patient care decisions based on sound reasoning in a more autonomous, less supervised fashion while caring for a much larger number of patients.

Hope's primary deficit was one of medical knowledge and clinical reasoning. The breadth of her medical knowledge was deemed inadequate for the requirements of her training level. Because of her inadequate knowledge base, she also had deficits in clinical reasoning, as she was unable to efficiently retrieve illness scripts, make key connections, or demonstrate adequate understanding of important physiological/medical concepts – especially in a time-pressured clinical scenario.

Hope's medical knowledge deficits also compounded her deficits in time management and organization. Because it took time for her to look up concepts (that her peers did not need to) while pre-rounding, she struggled to complete her work and appeared under-prepared during rounds.

During clinical rotations and on tests, Hope also faced anxiety about her performance that impacted her mental well-being. Because she had initially failed and retaken USMLE Step 1 during medical school, anticipating and preparing for her upcoming Step 3 exam created additional stress during her internship. Hope's awareness of her inadequate performance and fear of failure triggered an anxiety disorder previously diagnosed during medical school. For example, she would arrive to work at 5 AM to give herself more time to pre-round, only to stumble through presentations and not present key information that she had written down as anxiety hindered her performance.

REMEDIATION APPROACH

Hope was placed on a structured learning plan for medical knowledge and clinical reasoning beginning in the last 2 months of her PGY-1 year. The decision to initiate remediation was recommended to the program director by the residency program's clinical competency committee (CCC), a multi-disciplinary group of core teaching faculty tasked with reviewing feedback and evaluations on residents' performance and making recommendations to the residency program on implementing educational interventions, remediation, or disciplinary action. The remediation plan was developed by Hope's faculty advisor and the associate program director with input from the chair of the CCC. During the period of remediation, the faculty advisor met with Hope every two weeks to review and discuss her academic progress. The faculty advisor reported back to the CCC about Hope's progress monthly.

> Editor: In this, the 21st case, recurrent themes continue to emerge.
> **Delays in remediation** – While challenges were noted 6 months into Hope's internship, it took another 4 months to start remediation.
> **Medical knowledge as the foundation** – Without medical knowledge, one cannot develop skills in clinical reasoning, communication, time management and organization, professional development, and systems-based practice while maintaining a healthy sense of self.
> **Conflicts of interest** – If the associate program director is part of the remediation plan, then it should be made clear to the learner that the director will not participate in academic progress or status decisions. The learner needs to have a safe learning environment in which to make mistakes, ask questions, and reveal concerns to make progress.

Hope's initial remediation plan was scheduled for 6 months with a PGY-1 extension of 6 months. At the end of 6 months, the CCC deemed that Hope had achieved the goals of the medical knowledge portion of the remediation plan but required ongoing support and intervention to further improve her clinical reasoning skills. Using shared decision-making with Hope, who also believed she needed additional time to improve her clinical skills, the CCC decided to extend the remediation period for an additional 4 months with a focus on remediating clinical reasoning during the remaining months – although the resident had been promoted to the PGY-2 level during that time.

During the remediation period and the rest of her training, Hope proactively sought out resources and successfully addressed her anxiety. She found that working with her psychologist to receive cognitive behavioral therapy and meditation exercises were the most helpful. The counseling helped build her self-confidence as she was reminded of her successes and helped her formulate concrete strategies to not only manage her anxiety but also improve her time management, information gathering, and knowledge acquisition.

The following sections describe the specific strategies used for remediation of both medical knowledge and clinical reasoning. Note that the methods to assess progress in achieving learning goals were pre-defined at the outset of remediation.

Strategies Employed to Improve Medical Knowledge
For the medical knowledge portion of the remediation plan, Hope took an initial medical knowledge assessment test, a 100-question multiple-choice question test created by the CCC chair on a wide range of internal medicine questions. Her initial score was approximately 50%; she was then given an opportunity to review the questions and topics missed. With the aim of passing the test, Hope developed a 6-month long study plan to improve knowledge in her subject areas of weakness. Resources used for studying included Medical Knowledge Self-Assessment Program (MKSAP) books (bought by the program for communal use) and the *New England Journal of Medicine* (NEJM) Knowledge+ Online Question Bank (bought by the program and made available to all residents). Hope created a study plan with her faculty advisor's input that was realistic, goal-oriented, and prioritized to focus on areas of knowledge deficits defined by her performance on the initial diagnostic assessment test. Part of this plan included creating flashcards with illness scripts, including basic pathophysiology. The study plan was also individualized to match Hope's bandwidth during certain clinical rotations. During intense clinical rotations, her study goals were more limited, while her study goals were more comprehensive during less time-intensive rotations.

She reviewed thirteen subject areas and approximately 1300 questions in the NEJM Knowledge+ question bank over the course of six months. At the end of the remediation period, she re-took the initial Medical Knowledge Assessment Test with a passing score of >80%.

> *Editor: Pairing study topics with rotation subjects or patient cases can help with retention of material learned.[1] For example, the study plan could include reviewing the cardiology questions and cardiology review material while on her cardiology rotation and the pulmonary questions and pulmonary review material while on her ICU rotation. As questions arise with the respective content, faculty will be available to help answer queries and explain any areas of confusion.*
>
> *Many of our learners take notes on the computer. Information is better mastered and ingrained into memory if written by hand and reviewed by testing one's memory multiple times in recall fashion. Old-fashioned handwritten flashcards remain a great method for learning medical information.[2,3]*

In addition to studying resources, creating flashcards, and answering multiple-choice questions, Hope was directed to apply the medical knowledge she was acquiring to her clinical notes. For each note, she was asked to include 1-2 sentences about the pathophysiology guiding the most-likely differential diagnosis for her patients. This was implemented to apply her medical knowledge gained from reading to actual cases and patient encounters, with the goal of promoting both knowledge application and retention.

Strategies Employed to Improve Clinical Reasoning

There were two strategies employed to improve Hope's clinical reasoning. First, she worked one-on-one with several core faculty members on solving clinical cases. These cases were adapted from the *New England Journal of Medicine* Clinical Problem-Solving case series. They contain aliquots of data interspersed with deliberate breaks in which the resident is asked to discuss the case, provide a diagnostic framework for approaching a particular problem, and prioritize the top items on their differential diagnosis based on the information given. As the case progresses, the learner is asked to further refine their clinical reasoning based on new aliquots of data and defend any management decisions they might make. Initially, Hope completed these scenarios in writing, providing her with time to build diagnostic schemas and carefully think through the management in a non-time pressured way before submitting her answers to her faculty preceptor for review and feedback. Towards the end of the remediation period, Hope completed these cases orally (in person) with a faculty preceptor, requiring her to access illness scripts and articulate her reasoning approach in a time-pressured way as is often required in clinical practice. An example of a clinical solving case is included (see **Appendix B**).

Editor: Diagnostic schemas or decision-tree algorithms that the learner creates are conducive to learning clinical reasoning and aid coaches in providing feedback to their learners. The coach can see what is missing from the learner's thought process and where the learner got distracted or diverged from the correct cognitive path.[4,5]

Most learners learn best when verbal teaching is combined with visual learning, reading, and active learning such as writing or drawing. It is easy to incorporate multiple modalities as you are teaching to help the learner retain the pearls that they are learning. It also helps reduce miscommunication that can occur with verbal teaching alone.

The second strategy employed to improve clinical reasoning skills was to improve the frequency and quality of feedback Hope received on her reasoning skills during clinical rotations. She was asked to submit a "Clinical Reasoning Feedback Form" (see **Appendix C**) to attendings with whom she worked on both inpatient and ambulatory rotations to elicit more frequent and specific feedback on her clinical reasoning as evident in her notes and oral presentations. This strategy was employed with the intent to encourage other teaching faculty or preceptors to serve in a more active coaching role to support Hope's professional development in this domain.

DISCIPLINARY ACTION

Hope received remediation and extension of her PGY-1 year by 6 months, but no disciplinary actions were ever taken. After the completion of remediation, she completed the remainder of her training without any formal educational interventions.

Editor: If there are delays in academic progression of a learner, as in this case from PGY-1 to PGY-2 year, a letter of warning is recommended. It helps set the groundwork in case remediation does not go well and the program needs to move towards dismissal or contract non-renewal. It also formally justifies delay in progression in case she ever questions why she was being treated differently from other learners.

SUCCESSES

The feedback forms were an especially useful tool in this educational intervention. When the narrative comments included in these forms were specific and targeted towards making achievable changes, Hope was immediately able to adapt her practice and grow. She appreciated the detailed written feedback in these forms compared to traditional face-to-face feedback, as written comments allowed her time to introspect and internalize the feedback in her own time. This approach may work well for more introverted learners who value time to independently process information. In addition, Hope was most receptive to feedback from supervisors who established a safe learning environment with her; she understood that the purpose of corrective feedback from these individuals was to coach her to grow rather than to assign value judgments about her competency. Similarly, working through clinical reasoning cases with a faculty member created another opportunity for targeted feedback on her clinical reasoning skills and focus on her learning in an engaging case-based format.

From a programmatic perspective, feedback forms were useful for several reasons. First, the forms placed the responsibility of coaching and providing feedback widely on all teaching faculty rather than on an individual remediation coach. Because this program is a non-academic community hospital with limited resources, having dedicated faculty to serve as experienced remediation coaches separate from the CCC process was neither realistic nor achievable. The feedback forms promoted the provision of targeted and focused feedback within the resource-limited constraints of this residency program. Second, the return rates of these forms by faculty were much higher as compared to traditional, end-of-rotation evaluation form completion rates. Finally, the information contained in the feedback forms was useful to the CCC as sources of both formative assessment during remediation and as summative assessment at the end of remediation. The forms contained an abundance of information on the resident's performance to make even-handed and fair recommendations to continue, modify, or end remediation.

OPPORTUNITIES TO LEARN

The feedback forms also contained some limitations. Hope cited that certain attendings, when asked by her to fill out a feedback form, responded with exasperation, as though she was assigning them yet another task to complete. In these scenarios, Hope noted that "the process of asking for feedback became humiliating." Such experiences may discourage residents from seeking feedback in the future, which may hinder successful remediation. Second, Hope noted that the questions on the feedback form asking the supervisor to provide numeric ratings were less useful to her growth as compared to the free-form narrative comments.

HINDSIGHT REFLECTIONS FROM THE REMEDIATING FACULTY

Given that Hope cited opportunities to receive high-quality feedback as one of the most effective interventions in the remediation process, we have made the following changes to improve the remediation process. First, rather than ask the resident to submit feedback forms to her attendings, we ask a residency program administrator to email feedback forms weekly to specific attendings with whom the resident works, with the resident copied on these emails. Next, we have decreased the number of questions on the feedback form requiring numerical rating answers, and instead ask the supervisor to focus on providing high-quality written/narrative feedback citing examples and observed behaviors. Finally, we have implemented semi-annual faculty development sessions on how to provide effective written and verbal feedback.

The second change that would have supported Hope's growth more effectively would have been to give her more of a voice in shaping the remediation plan. One of the reasons why this intervention was successful was because Hope had insight and skills in self-regulated learning. As such, she indicated that she would have appreciated more input in certain elements of the process – including choosing her faculty advisor and mentors as well as some degree of clinical schedule flexibility to support her independent study to acquire more medical knowledge. Incorporating the learner's suggestions and enabling some degree of reasonable flexibility with the remediation plan is ideal for adult learners.

Finally, Hope indicated that program-wide interventions to de-stigmatize the remediation process would be helpful. Noon conferences or academic time dedicated to honest discussion of academic remediation, as well as stories of learners who had gone through the remediation process and who are now successfully practicing medicine would help normalize the experience and potentially mitigate the shame and anxiety that invariably comes with the process. The program plans to incorporate this into the curriculum.

Editor: When working with struggling learners, the editor spends a considerable amount of time talking about the process – mostly to alleviate anxiety and fear as most learners think that they will be fired the next day. Beyond the individual learner, when a struggling learner continues to visibly struggle, enters remediation, repeats a year, takes time off, or is dismissed from a program, other residents may question whether the program is doing anything to help – and they question the security of their own position in the residency program. Even though information about the struggling learner is disseminated on a need-to-know basis only, that doesn't mean that the topic should be avoided. Program directors and designated institutional officers (DIOs) should talk to residents and fellows with the goal of destigmatizing remediation by explaining the process, how it differs from disciplinary action, that it takes time and works better with peer support, how disciplinary action and due process works at the institution, and how to seek academic, physical, and mental health support. 🖗

REFERENCES

1   Artemeva N, Rachul C, O'Brien B, Varpio L. Situated learning in medical education. *Acad Med.* 2017 Jan 1;92(1):134.

2   Smoker TJ, Murphy CE, Rockwell AK. Comparing memory for handwriting versus typing. Proceedings of the Human Factors and Ergonomics Society Annual Meeting 2009 Oct (Vol. 53, No. 22, pp. 1744-1747). Sage CA: Los Angeles, CA: SAGE Publications.

3   Cooke NM, Durso FT, Schvaneveldt RW. Recall and measures of memory organization. *Journal of Experimental Psychology: Learning, Memory, and Cognition.* 1986 Oct;12(4):538.

4   Guerrasio J, Aagaard EM. Methods and outcomes for the remediation of clinical reasoning. *JGIM.* 2014 Dec 1;29(12):1607-14.

5   Higgs J, Jones MA, Loftus S, Christensen N, editors. *Clinical Reasoning in the Health Professions* E-book. Elsevier Health Sciences; 2008 Feb 18.

CASE 22

Time Management and Organization and Clinical Reasoning

LEARNER AT TIME OF IDENTIFICATION FOR REMEDIATION

Leenor, a third-month, first post-graduate year resident in internal medicine

REASON FOR REMEDIATION

Leenor was an international medical graduate who attended medical school in Asia prior to starting his internal medicine residency in the U.S (after a three-year gap). Though over 34,000 international medical graduates (IMGs) matched into U.S. residency programs in 2020, and they comprise 25% of the physician workforce, their experiences are not often represented in the medical literature on remediation. Like many IMGs, Leenor had taken time off between completing medical school and starting internship. The gap between medical school and residency (largely unavoidable given the requirements of transitioning from a non-U.S. school) as well as the language and cultural differences presented him with significant adjustment challenges – in addition to the usual challenges that all new interns face.

At the start of his intern year, Leenor encountered the immediate demands of learning to manage his pager, navigate the hospital, and use three different electronic medical record systems. He had "sky high anxiety" when he received new pages and felt unprepared for the high reliance on technology demanded by the U.S. medical system. The challenges of an unfamiliar healthcare system were compounded by the fast pace and high volume of patient care in a U.S. hospital. He was unable to prioritize tasks, often missed gathering data, and was not reliable in completing tasks. He required close supervision by his supervisors to ensure patient-care tasks were completed on time.

Leenor also faced a new set of expectations related to the format of rounding, the structure of presentations, the communication of clinical reasoning, and new documentation conventions in the U.S. medical system, all of which differed from his prior medical training. His presentations were not consistently organized in the traditional SOAP format and he often missed pertinent data despite their lengthiness. During medical school, he was accustomed to carrying out his attendings' plans unquestioningly, rather than being expected to formulate his plans independently and justify them with clinical reasoning. His attendings in residency noted that his presentations sometimes ended abruptly after he presented the objective data, as he was unsure of how to create and express his own assessment and plan. Attendings at times perceived this behavior as a lack of ownership of his patients or disinterest in helping advance the care of his patients. They often had to repeat the work of obtaining a complete history and physical exam as he was completely reliant on them to formulate a plan.

Leenor's deficits were primarily in time management and organization and clinical reasoning. Initially, he was thought to have deficits in medical knowledge due to his challenges with creating his own assessment and plan, formulating a differential diagnosis, and building a clinical argument based on supporting evidence. But over time he demonstrated good recall of disease pathophysiology, diagnosis, and management.

Editor: This is a remarkable summary of just some of the challenges faced by our IMG residents, and it doesn't even address the psychosocial issues associated with being away from one's home, family and friends, language, and culture. What we know about IMGs who have worked so hard to study and take USMLE exams to get into American residencies is that they are resilient, dedicated, and teachable, despite having mountains more to learn than their American-trained peers. One can only hope that there are other IMG residents, ideally from the same culture, that can help support them, share comaradery, and provide useful tips and tricks that they have learned along the way.

REMEDIATION APPROACH

Leenor was placed on a 3-month remediation plan for time management and organization and clinical reasoning. The decision to initiate remediation was recommended to the program director by the residency program's clinical competency committee (CCC), a multi-disciplinary group of core teaching faculty tasked with reviewing feedback and evaluations on residents' performance and making recommendations to the residency program on implementing educational interventions, remediation, or disciplinary action. The remediation plan was developed by the resident's faculty advisor and the associate program director with input from the CCC chair. During the period of remediation, the faculty advisor met with Leenor every two weeks to review and discuss his academic progress and provide coaching. The faculty advisor gave monthly reports to the CCC on Leenor's progress.

The following sections describe the specific strategies used for remediation of both time management and organization and clinical reasoning. Note that the methods to assess progress in achieving learning goals were pre-defined at the outset of remediation.

Strategies Employed to Improve Time Management and Organization

Leenor received information on strategies to improve his time management and organizational skills, including his institution's time management and organization resource sheet. (See **Appendix D**) This resource provides concrete advice on how much time to spend during wards completing various common aspects of an intern's workflow, such as pre-rounding on the computer and seeing patients before rounds. It offers recommendations on how to prioritize tasks during each phase of the day (pre-rounding, rounds, and afternoons) to complete tasks such that the most time-sensitive and important tasks are accomplished first, while minimizing disruptions to the intern's workflow. It also offers organization tips such as using a task list sheet to manage and track completion of all patient care tasks.

Editor: In addition to the resource sheet, a remediator or chief resident should go side-by-side with Leenor through an entire day and show him how to most efficiently utilize the electronic record, pre-round, organize paperwork, and complete tasks that need to be sequenced throughout his day. Leenor walked into a world without knowing the expectations, and he needs someone to review them with him in both inpatient and outpatient settings. The first step of providing feedback is setting the expectations.[1,2]

To offer additional advice, a chief resident observed Leenor using the resource sheet while pre-rounding on a few occasions. Leenor received feedback and coaching on the efficiency of his workflow and suggestions for improvement. Use of a near-peer mentor such as a chief resident can often be helpful as they may share highly specific advice for navigating the system smoothly and accessing resources more easily, including aspects of system-based practice of which even attendings may not be aware.

While incorporating the advice from the resource sheet and chief residents, Leenor improved his time management skills primarily through timing himself while doing common tasks throughout the day. To try to shorten the time required for each task, he used his cellphone to set a timer when pre-rounding in the morning on wards, during patient visits in clinic, or while giving case presentations to his attendings. Over this iterative process, he was able to optimize his time management such that he was accomplishing the objectives of each task in less time than previously required. With greater efficiency in his pre-rounding workflow, he had more time to focus on formulating a plan before rounds.

Strategies Employed to Improve Clinical Reasoning

To improve the frequency and quality of feedback he received on his presentation skills during clinical rotations, Leenor was asked to submit an oral presentation feedback form (see **Appendix E**) to attendings he worked with on both inpatient and ambulatory rotations. The form asks his supervisors to assess his ability to adhere to the expected order of information for the presentation, present information within a reasonable time frame, have a prioritized problem list that integrates pertinent data, and create a reasonable differential diagnosis for each active problem. Similarly, for his ambulatory patient care skills, he was required to obtain at least 5 clinic observation feedback forms from attendings which asked similar questions.

This allowed Leenor to receive real-time and targeted feedback on specific elements of his oral presentations and clinical reasoning process.

The written feedback forms were submitted by Leenor to his faculty advisor during their bi-weekly meetings. This provided his advisor with written information on his performance and additional data for coaching.

Editor: Without knowing more, there are many reasons to be hopeful about this resident. He just needs a chance to learn the new expectations, and there is a very good chance he will succeed, though his growth curve will be slower, and remediation is still warranted. Don't just tell him the expectations. Demonstrate them.

Remediation would have been much quicker if, before beginning on-site clinical feedback, Leenor had been given more direct upfront clinical reasoning teaching and structured cases to practice as described in previous cases. But this demonstrates that there are many ways to be successful with remediation as long as 3 components are included in the plan: practice, feedback, and reflection – followed by more practice, feedback and reflection.[3]

DISCIPLINARY ACTION

The resident's initial structured learning plan was intended for 3 months, but scores on his evaluation forms at the conclusion of the 3-month period did not meet the targets set by the initial remediation plan. When Leenor continued to demonstrate deficits in time management, organization, and clinical reasoning despite ongoing feedback and coaching, he was escalated to probation, and his intern year was extended by 6 months. While he was on academic probation, he started to make significant improvement in his clinical performance with ongoing intensive feedback and coaching. He was ultimately taken off probation and resumed a second structured learning plan for 3 additional months (later extended to 6 months) to improve his management plans in the ambulatory setting. Leenor was able to achieve the goals of this remediation plan and thus was advanced to his second year of residency after 15 months of internship training. He completed the remainder of his training without any formal educational interventions. In fact, he exceeded expectations in several milestone areas and was recommended for and successfully matched into a subspecialty medicine fellowship.

SUCCESSES

Addressing the time management and organizational concerns first was an effective strategy as it freed up more time for Leenor to practice the steps of clinical reasoning. Using a near peer to offer specific time-saving strategies for efficiency helped build upon the time management advice in the resource sheet. What Leenor found most helpful for addressing the clinical reasoning concerns were the feedback forms. He appreciated receiving feedback in a timely manner from a wide range of attendings who could offer suggestions on different aspects of his performance.

OPPORTUNITIES TO LEARN

Escalating Leenor's remediation plan to probation was not an effective educational strategy. The perception of his performance as passive and lacking engagement around clinical decision-making may have led the institution to escalate to probation too soon. In fact, his apparent disengagement was likely due to his significant discomfort and guardedness about practicing medicine in a new cultural context, rather than apathy toward patient care. Placing him on probation likely exacerbated the sense of his status as a cultural outsider and contributed to his existing performance challenges. Leenor felt that being placed on probation further depleted his already low confidence.

> *Editor: As mentioned earlier, if there are delays in progression of a learner, if not probation, a letter of warning, at the very least, is recommended. It helps set the groundwork in case remediation does not go well and the program needs to move towards dismissal or contract non-renewal. A warning letter also formally justifies delay in progression in case the learner ever questions why he was being treated differently from other learners. This also provides the program with some legal protection. At the same time, it does demoralize some residents. Perhaps a warning would have been less harsh than probation. Let the remediator remain the "good person" and the program director be the "bad person" who carries out the recommendations of the CCC, so as not to ruin the working relationship between the remediator and the learner.*

Hindsight Reflections from the Remediating Faculty

We believe there are several interventions that could have helped facilitate this learner's transition to internship in the U.S. before and during his training.

Based on our experience working with Leenor and other IMGs, our program has since implemented a more extensive set of orientation activities for IMG interns. Whereas Leenor underwent a one-day IMG orientation, we now offer IMG interns the option to shadow in the hospital and clinics for up to two weeks prior to the start of internship to help familiarize them with the electronic medical record (EMR) and hospital system as well as observe rounds and delivery of patient care in a low-stakes situation. We use a peer mentorship system in which new IMG interns are paired with an IMG resident who can help reduce the sense of culture shock and facilitate acculturation. Finally, we distribute the time management and organization resource sheet to all interns at the start of their training to help them transition to their new role.

In terms of other pre-work, sending learners some suggested study resources to review prior to starting their internships could help them refresh their medical knowledge – particularly for learners who have taken time off from clinical roles before starting residency. Connecting learners with a faculty mentor even prior to internship can help establish trust and set expectations for resident performance early. During orientation, small group sessions discussing professional expectations for physicians can also help set expectations created and reinforced by the residents themselves to emphasize shared values and foster professional identity formation.

Creating an inclusive learning climate and offering frequent, timely, and specific feedback throughout residency is essential for all learners, particularly IMGs who often face stigma associated with their background in academic settings. Common practices in academic medicine, such as team introductions that rely on self-identification of prior institutions of training, may inadvertently create an environment in which IMGs may feel excluded. Implicit bias training among faculty should be prioritized and targeted towards considering the needs of IMGs – who make up a considerable part of the healthcare force. Their particular needs are often overlooked, but there are challenges such as stereotype threat that they share with struggling residents from underrepresented minority backgrounds. We intend to build faculty development opportunities to familiarize attendings with tools to create an inclusive, positive learning climate and help learners of all backgrounds feel heard and comfortably challenged. ⌭

REFERENCES

1   Stone D, Heen S. *Thanks for the feedback: The science and art of receiving feedback well (even when it is off base, unfair, poorly delivered, and frankly, you're not in the mood).* Penguin; 2015.

2   Hewson MG, Little ML. Giving feedback in medical education: verification of recommended techniques. *JGIM.* 1998 Feb;13(2):111-6.

3   Warburton KM, Goren E, Dine CJ. Comprehensive assessment of struggling learners referred to a graduate medical education remediation program. *JGME.* 2017 Dec;9(6):763-7.

CASE 23

Mental Well-Being, Professionalism, Medical Knowledge, Clinical Reasoning, and Interpersonal skills

LEARNER AT TIME OF IDENTIFICATION FOR REMEDIATION

Jenny, a second post-graduate year resident in emergency medicine (three-year program)

REASON FOR REMEDIATION

At the beginning of her PGY-2 year, Jenny suffered a noticeable decline in her functioning as an emergency medicine resident. She was distracted while working, regardless of the task or who she was working with. This was clearly a deterioration from her level of competency at the end of her PGY-1 year. She presented patient cases with incomplete information, both in history gathering and physical exam findings. She was not able to develop a relevant differential diagnosis and did not demonstrate understanding of the conditions of the patients she was managing. The faculty noticed and verbalized to the program director an eroding trust in her performing entrustable professional activities. On two occasions Jenny began crying and had to leave the ED when challenged by the faculty that her performance was not meeting expectations. Her medical knowledge as reported by the faculty was below expectations and she scored in the first percentile on the yearly in-training examination. In addition, her interpersonal skills regressed, and she would not make eye-contact with attending physicians, consultants, or other residents.

> *Editor: Acute declines in performance are almost always related to the category of mental well-being and may more specifically be from a new medical diagnosis, a chronic medical condition that is now uncontrolled, a new psychiatric disorder, a chronic psychiatric condition that is now uncontrolled, or a new life stress. The conditions range from a new brain tumor or abscess, to a psychotic break, to a change in medication, to sleep deprivation, a dying parent, or marital strife.*

REMEDIATION APPROACH

Following the methods from the book *Remediation of the Struggling Medical Learner*, all deficiencies were not remediated simultaneously. Rather, a targeted approach to address the primary deficiency was taken first, with subsequent deficiencies to be addressed if/when the more pressing deficiency was remediated. The residency program director (PD), with the guidance of the clinical competency committee (CCC), designed and led the remediation strategies.

Remediation Strategy #1: Mental Well-being
After multiple meetings discussing her struggles, it was identified that Jenny had unresolved social barriers affecting her performance. She identified strained social/romantic relationships and strained familial relationships along with financial and residential/housing uncertainties as barriers to her ability to function as a resident. She confirmed that she was physically safe in her relationships and current housing. She denied any substance abuse or even use, and none was suspected based on her behavior. She was not willing to provide details into her strained relationships and struggles. She also could not identify which was the most prominent nor the actual effects each had on her performance.

> *Editor: Part of the reason that Jenny was not willing to provide details is because her program director was directly involved in her remediation. As with prior cases, program directors care a tremendous amount about their learners, but that can be difficult for learners to see since they serve several*

> *roles – including carrying out the recommendations of the CCC. Program*
> *directors cannot create a truly safe learning environment no matter how*
> *hard they try. It is inherent in the role that they play.*[1,2]

The PD mandated that Jenny make an appointment to see a psychologist/therapist for a single visit because she identified an inability to reconcile her personal/home life and professional obligations at this time. Jenny was offended by the mandate but agreed as part of her remediation plan.

Within 4 weeks of initiating therapy, Jenny began presenting herself with a confident posture, re-initiated eye-contact when in conversation, and her crying episodes in the department resolved.

After initiating counseling sessions with a therapist, Jenny's mental well-being, professionalism (crying during ER shifts), and interpersonal skills deficiencies were resolved.

Remediation Strategy #2: Medical Knowledge
Participating in therapy helped Jenny reconcile, if not resolve, her mental well-being struggles. However, she was still functioning below expectations in her demonstration of medical knowledge and clinical reasoning during ER shifts. Additionally, she scored in the first percentile of all residents taking the yearly in-training exam. In questioning this, she stated that anxiety was crippling her ability to demonstrate her medical knowledge. She stated that she stared at the front page of the in-training exam for the first 45 minutes of the exam, too anxious to even get started, which in turn resulted in being unable to finish the exam in the allotted time. She identified experiencing social anxiety, specific to those in a supervisory role, that was noticeable when presenting cases to attendings. It prevented her from relaying important aspects of the patient cases.

Since anxiety was identified as directly inhibiting her ability to function, the remediation strategy was for Jenny to see a psychiatrist to determine if her anxiety could be treated.

She agreed to see a psychiatrist. She did not provide details of the encounter, but she relayed that after a single visit the psychiatrist determined that her anxiety did not meet the level of a mental illness and that psychiatric intervention was not needed nor would be beneficial for her. No further psychiatric interventions were recommended or pursued.

Remediation Strategy #2: Medical Knowledge – Take 2

Editor: Before moving on, roadblocks are common in remediation. Not every strategy will work. Sometimes the diagnosis needs to be reevaluated. Sometimes the learner isn't as cooperative as we would like for them to be. Other times those we hope would help, such as the psychiatrist in this case, are less than helpful. To give the psychiatrist the benefit of the doubt, perhaps Jenny didn't disclose enough information for the psychiatrist to see her true level of anxiety. Maybe the psychiatrist completely missed the diagnosis. Or the psychiatrist may have recommended a plan that Jenny did not agree with. Say Jenny was opposed to the medication recommended and found it easier to report that no intervention was recommended. When a strategy does not work, either reassess the diagnosis or try a new strategy. Instead of getting reports from the learner, ask the learner to sign a release so the remediator can speak to the psychiatrist directly. This will ensure that the information that the program wants the psychiatrist to know gets communicated as well as the psychiatrist's recommendations.

Having eliminated psychiatric issues as a barrier to her demonstrating requisite medical knowledge, the PD met with Jenny to identify topics she, herself, felt were deficient in her medical knowledge. The goal of this approach was to engage Jenny under the principles of adult learning and to reinforce practice-based learning skills. An individualized learning plan to include a structured reading curriculum, to be completed on top of the requisite readings for all residents, was designed by the resident. The PD scheduled follow-up meetings to discuss the material.

Editor: Several cases have given struggling learners the ability to contribute to their remediation plan. This helps establish buy-in, allows the learner to assess what they think is a feasible amount of work, and promotes self-directed learning.[3]

Reading alone is too passive. The remediation plan in this case includes topic discussions which help the learner move into an active phase that allows for deeper understanding and retention. Answering questions along with reading can serve a similar function, as it is more active than reading alone.

After three meetings to discuss the material, the PD noticed that Jenny had a strong grasp of the reading material. In discussing this with her, she iterated that she understands the material well, but her ability to apply and present the knowledge is lacking. It was agreed upon to discontinue the structured reading curriculum because of the large time-burden on the resident and because it was not directly addressing the deficiency.

Remediation Strategy #3: Clinical Reasoning
Jenny's ability to retain medical knowledge was not deficient, but her ability to apply and present the knowledge was lacking. In designing the next step in the remediation plan, Jenny and the PD scheduled individual sessions with multiple different faculty, deliberately including faculty that Jenny identified as intimidating and/or making her nervous. During these sessions, pre-identified topics would be discussed. The faculty would provide case-based scenarios requiring Jenny to apply and present her medical knowledge. These 1 to 2-hour sessions were held every other week for 12 weeks. During these low-stakes, low-stress, psychologically safe environments, Jenny became more comfortable and confident in applying and demonstrating her medical knowledge to the faculty. This translated well to her becoming more comfortable and confident in presenting actual patient cases to the same attending physicians in the high-stakes, high-stress emergency department environment.

As a result of these interventions, by the middle of her PGY-3 year, Jenny's ability to gather and relay relevant patient information, to demonstrate understanding of the conditions of the patients she was managing, to perform entrustable professional activities, and to demonstrate medical knowledge all significantly improved. She was able to appropriately manage multiple critical/ high stress patients competently. While she was still performing below her peers after the remediation strategies, she was no longer deemed deficient in these areas by the clinical competency committee. Her formal individualized learning plan was determined resolved and lifted.

Jenny was considered by the clinical competency committee and program director to be competent in emergency medicine and able to practice safely and independently upon graduation.

DISCIPLINARY ACTION

No disciplinary actions were taken. Jenny was highly motivated to improve and willingly followed all remediation plans, even when she did not necessarily agree with the plan.

SUCCESSES

Several factors made this a successful endeavor:

1. Jenny had insight that there was a problem. She herself wasn't clear as to what the problem(s) was, but she realized that there was a problem, and she was motivated to participate in strategies to address her deficiencies.
2. The program director (with the guidance of the clinical competency committee) stuck to the strategy of remediating one deficiency at a time and did not try to fix all problems simultaneously.
3. The program director and Jenny were both patient when remediation strategies didn't work, remained undeterred, and were willing to try other strategies.
4. Jenny had a strong support network from her fellow residents. Although the remediation plan was never discussed with other residents, it was well-known that she was struggling. At the beginning of the remediation process, she confided in her colleagues that she felt that the program leadership and the program director were abandoning her and laying the groundwork to remove her from the program. This led to thoughts of despair on her part, resulting in her fellow residents checking in frequently on her well-being. This also led to communication from other residents to the program director offering their support of her and, some with hostility, criticizing the program director for being too harsh with her. The program director was comforted knowing that Jenny had a group of colleagues caring and advocating for her. About mid-way through the remediation process, Jenny's perspective changed, and she acknowledged the efforts of the program director and faculty in their support and dedication to her success.

Jenny graduated on time, having successfully completed her remediation plans and meeting all qualifications of completing the residency. Upon graduation she was performing below her peers but demonstrating competency and ability to safely provide emergency medical care. Equally important, she was happy and carried herself with pride and confidence.

OPPORTUNITIES TO LEARN

Several lessons were learned in referring residents to therapy:

1. Although Jenny was reluctant at first to see a therapist, the therapist turned out to be a tremendous benefit to her; she continued to see the therapist twice per month long after her remediation was resolved. Her seeing a therapist was so much more beneficial than was ever anticipated.
2. Once they began offering, referring, or recommending the option for therapy to residents during semi-annual evaluations, the program was surprised as to how many residents wanted to participate in therapy but would not initiate unless recommended or offered.
3. There is no right approach to helping residents establish a therapist. Some residents expressed a desire for therapy, but a passive approach to simply provide them with resources often lead to residents not following through and scheduling appointments. For other residents, the program was more prescriptive in finding/assigning a therapist, only to have that patient/therapist relationship not work-out – causing the resident to have to go to lengths to find a different therapist. The residents made the dating analogy: not every patient and therapist work together and finding the right therapist is a personal decision/ endeavor. The best approach found was to simply ask the resident how involved he/she wants me to be in helping them establish a therapist, then engage in the level that the resident desires.

HINDSIGHT REFLECTIONS FROM THE REMEDIATING FACULTY

Jenny's deficiencies were so severe, and progress so limited initially that we honestly thought that successful remediation would not be possible. In the spirit of transparency, in frequent communications with her, we tried to balance support for her with conveying the expectation that if she did not improve, she would not be able to graduate from the program. While we thought we communicated well, the feedback from what she was telling other residents was that we were not creating a supportive environment for her. In fact, she felt like we were abandoning her and initiating the process to remove her from the program. During subsequent meetings, and her tremendous improvement and resolution of multiple deficiencies, she stated she felt more supported. But the lesson learned is that while clear communication with expectations is essential, the delivery of the message could have been tempered to better ensure support was communicated clearly.

> *Editor: The editor believes in direct and honest communication. The message doesn't need to be tempered. It just needs to come from the PD with someone else providing the remediation so as not to lose the trusting and collaborative relationship that is necessary between the remediator and the learner.*[4] 🗩

REFERENCES

1   Kalet A, Chou CL, Ellaway RH. To fail is human: remediating remediation in medical education. *Perspect Med Educ.* 2017;6:418-24.

2   Kebaetse MB, Winston K. Physician remediation: accepting and working with complementary conceptualisations. *Med Educ.* 2019;53:210-1.

3   Chou CL, Kalet A, Costa MJ, et al. Guidelines: The dos, don'ts and don't knows of remediation in medical education. *Perspect Med Educ.* 2019;8:322-338.

4   Bennion LD, Durning SJ, LaRochelle J, et al. Untying the Gordian knot: remediation problems in medical schools that need remediation. *BMC Med Educ.* 2018;18:120.

CASE 24

Clinical Reasoning, Time Management and Organization, Communication, Medical Knowledge, and Mental Well-Being

LEARNER AT TIME OF IDENTIFICATION FOR REMEDIATION

Jane, a second post-graduate year resident in obstetrics and gynecology

REASON FOR REMEDIATION

Jane was having difficulty functioning with others, as she did not communicate well with members of her team. In addition, she did not seem to understand feedback – nor was she able to apply it to patient care. She was also hypersensitive to criticism. Jane would try to change her behavior to please each faculty member, leading to more dysfunction as she tried to predict what each person wanted.

It was clear that Jane needed to acquire more knowledge, but she didn't know which topics to start learning first. She had difficulty prioritizing what basic knowledge to study. She also had difficulty applying her medical knowledge in clinical practice.

REMEDIATION APPROACH

Jane's remediation plan was designed using the following objectives:

- Apply standard feedback by pointing out the deficiencies and expectations for correcting those shortcomings over six months.

  Editor: The number of Jane's deficits is overwhelming. The editor might not present all of them to her at once, or would at least package them as 1 or 2 main problems that are leading to problems in other areas of her performance. Then emphasize that fixing 1 or 2 issues will help the others. Jane is already defensive. Try not to further demoralize her; propose the deficits in a way that addressing them seems manageable and not overwhelming.1

- Identify the specific ways in which Jane processes information differently from her peers. Use the Myers-Briggs Type Indicator as a tool to facilitate discussion.
- Limit teaching faculty to a small group of educators and evaluators for Jane to work with initially, before expanding to the rest of the faculty.
- Identify the difficulty Jane has in interpreting information from the environment and provide guidance for expanding her perception.

To improve her knowledge base, Jane was first asked to perform additional reading and then to discuss specific topics with faculty. This was not successful. When she was given penalties for lack of timeliness, this was not successful. Next, she was given increased time in the simulation lab. This was also not successful.

  Editor: Penalties usually don't work. Most learners want to do their best and don't want to get in trouble. If they had the tools to avoid getting in trouble, they would use them. Penalties don't work because they don't teach learners how to behave differently. They just add stress to an already stressful situation. Say for example you have a learner who is always late to afternoon clinic, so you propose a penalty if they are late in the future. Now instead of being late, they skip lunch or leave their morning clinical duties unfulfilled to avoid being late in the afternoon. Without new skills, this only creates a new problem.

Upon completing a Myers-Briggs Type Indicator questionnaire, one is given some indication as to what their personality preferences are in 4 domains:

extroversion versus introversion, sensing versus intuition, thinking versus feeling, and judging versus perceiving. This characterization helps people better understand their own learning preferences – and how others learn and receive information differently from them. The differences may pertain to various learning processes such as general interest, motivation factors, perceiving and comprehending the information, prioritizing, recollecting information, responding to feedback, and translating the data into a plan of action.

It is well known that the learning process is most effective when it is in line with learners' style preferences. Although there is little application of this dogma in postgraduate education, it makes intuitive sense that faculty personality preferences should play an essential role in modeling and training of residents. Hence, it is useful to know which learning methods are the most effective to help them acquire knowledge quickly and effectively. In this case, Jane's learning style conflicted with most of the faculty's Myers-Briggs preferences.

As determined by her Myers-Briggs testing, Jane's interest in learning is related to the question, "Will this help me work with others?" The more positive the answer to this question, the greater her interest in the topic – and the greater her desire to actively engage and apply what she learns. Students like Jane learn better when the material is people-oriented rather than strictly theoretical. They do not need the information to be logical to grasp it; they memorize details and learn better when their emotions are involved. In this personality type, constructive criticism tends to be taken negatively and perceived as a personal threat.

It became apparent that Jane was interested in studying something when she could see the possibility of gaining new skills and putting them into practice. Merely watching procedures deterred her interest in learning. She perceived this approach as a poor reflection of her abilities rather than an opportunity to learn. She retained new information when she devoted the topic's relevance to people – in this case, directed to the attending faculty rather than the patients.

Jane's learning preference allowed her to take in a substantial amount of information, but it lacked significant logical flow. That is why she had difficulty prioritizing which vital information needed to be known. Once her feelings and emotions were engaged, she was able to remember new material.

And when she received positive feedback, she began putting forth more effort.

Due to Jane's extroverted preference, she was often found to be thinking out loud, expressing various ideas before reaching a conclusion. An unaware, introverted faculty member misinterpreted this communication style as either belligerent or as showing a reasoning deficit.

Successful communication was achieved when the conversation began by showing concern for Jane's feelings and pointing to the faculty's feelings regarding patient care. Progress was made by showing Jane how the remediation correlated positively with her goals and how her action could impact people. She was coached that constructive criticism was not meant to degrade her, but it was a tool designed for self-improvement. She was educated about differences in teaching and feedback style among the faculty. She discovered the value of self-improvement and realized that she need not please everyone to be an accomplished person.

Jane currently enjoys learning and actively participates in lectures. She eagerly instructs students, taking pride in her knowledge. She still struggles with various attending personality preferences, but she is aware of the differences and is keenly working toward acceptance.

When it was recognized that she was living alone, far away from her family and friends, Jane reached out to the local community and church. She took the initiative to find a "life coach" to listen and mentor her through the self-improvement process. With the faculty and Jane's own understanding of her learning process, this was a remediation success for the resident and residency program.

Editor: Many learners see themselves as the benchmark of normalcy. They think that their perception of the world is the most accurate and the best way to approach learning, communication, interpersonal skills, and professionalism, among other things. It is very helpful for learners to understand that based on innate personality characteristics, others perceive and approach medicine very differently – while being just as effective. Those with seemingly opposing styles have a tremendous amount to teach us. They can expand our understanding of the world and add new tools and strategies to our toolbox. With this mature understanding and appreciation for diversity of thought processes, some of the most productive teams have members with different Myers-Briggs personality preferences.

DISCIPLINARY ACTION

Jane was placed on remediation, then probation, before successful completion of the process. Probation seemed to relate the seriousness of the concerns and allowed time for her to make changes.

SUCCESSES

The standard feedback did not achieve the desired effect. Jane perceived constructive criticism as a personal attack. The turning point was when the feedback approach was changed to match her Myers-Briggs personality preference, which included processing information, reaching conclusions, and reacting to the environment. The faculty was educated about Jane's interpretation of their feedback.

> *Editor: Any tool or framing of feedback that removes judgement from feedback will make it much more successful and better received. Make suggestions for what the learner should try next time they are in a similar situation to see if the outcome is different. Then talk through how the new strategy worked. Find tools like the Myers-Briggs test that normalize variability and discuss when to lean on different aspects of our personalities or skills. Make sure the scenarios for using the new strategies are very specifically defined.[1,2]*

HINDSIGHT REFLECTIONS FROM THE REMEDIATING FACULTY

We wish we had recognized Jane's deficiencies earlier and implemented a personalized study plan sooner, as well as noted her inability to take in constructive criticism as an intern. We should have educated the faculty about a different way to provide feedback and taught Jane about cognitive behavior thinking.

REFERENCES

1   Guerrasio J. *Remediation of the Struggling Medical Learner, 2nd Ed.* Irwin, PA: Association for Hospital Medical Education; 2017.

2   Stone D, Heen S. *Thanks for the feedback: The science and art of receiving feedback well (even when it is off base, unfair, poorly delivered, and frankly, you're not in the mood).* Penguin; 2015.

Summary and Final Thoughts

So many rich and valuable experiences have been conveyed in all the cases generously contributed by multiple authors from around the world and across various disciplines. Each example is filled with tips at various stages in the remediation process, and there is always something to learn – whether or not the learner succeeded in promotion or graduation. A brief summary cannot do the rich stories justice, but here are several key points that emerged, categorized by theme.

IDENTIFICATION

- Many programs wished that they had identified the struggling learner earlier or had initiated remediation plans sooner.
- Most struggling learners had multiple educational deficits.
- To diminish risks of bias, many cases obtained observations from multiple sources when identifying and diagnosing the struggling learner.

DIAGNOSIS

- Identifying all the learner's educational deficits accurately is key to successful remediation.
- It is important to clarify the learner's educational deficits with examples.

- It can be less overwhelming and more manageable to isolate the largest deficit – or at least the most significant deficits – which can then be targeted for remediation.
- External evaluations when indicated should include both physical and mental health examinations.
- Though you are comfortable using medical vernacular to describe your observations, remember that you are not your learner's clinician.

CHARACTERISTICS OF STRUGGLING LEARNERS

- Struggling learners are notoriously poor self-assessors.
- Learners who appear to lack insight need help receiving and implementing feedback.
- Struggling learners don't learn from the hidden curriculum. They need to be told directly what you would prefer they do.
- Struggling learners lack flexibility in applying their skills from one environment to the next.

FEEDBACK

- Start by setting clear expectations or clarifying previously stated expectations.
- Implement the key tenets of effective feedback (timely, behavior-based, based on observation, direct, clear, specific).
- Take judgement out of feedback by teaching learners how to ask for feedback.
- Role model how to accept feedback by receiving feedback on the remediation process and plan.

REMEDIATION

- Remediation plans must contain deliberate practice, feedback, and guided reflection.
- Consider including the learner in the design of the remediation plan.
- Remediation plans must be active rather than passive.
- Remediation plans must address how to accomplish the learning goals, not just what needs to be achieved.
- Identify your learner's motivation and begin remediation even if the learner doesn't yet possess insight.

- Utilize all modes of learning when teaching: reading, seeing, hearing, and actively doing.
- Remember that successful remediation takes patience and time and is truly a step-by-step process.
- Don't forget to reassess the learner to make sure that remediation was successful.

DISCIPLINE

- Clearly define and make known to the learner who makes disciplinary decisions and who carries out these decisions, as this should be someone other than the remediator(s).
- While there are no guidelines as to when to put a learner on probation or issue a letter of warning, consider doing so if the length of training is delayed, extended, or if you have concerns about a graduating learner.

INFRASTRUCTURE

- Remediation teams were often used for the benefit of shared knowledge, experience, expertise, and sharing of remediation responsibilities.
- Several programs reported having centralized remediation programs for their institution or at least one person with experience on each remediation team.
- Strongly consider feeding information forward to those who can help with the remediation process. Be sure to let the learner know what and with whom the information is being shared.
- Work to destigmatize remediation and make clear that it is not a disciplinary action.
- Educate all your faculty, house staff, and students on the process of remediation and disciplinary actions.
- When building your remediation infrastructure, remediation should not be conducted by anyone who has or might be perceived as having a conflict of interest (i.e., someone who evaluates or makes promotion decisions about the learner).
- Provide guidance to faculty and program leadership on the needed documentation, review and update policies, and understand the due process for your institution.
- Get to know your legal counsel before situations become urgent, have

them readily available, and make use of them.
- Provide diversity and inclusion training for remediation faculty.
- Make a list of all local resources that might assist with remediation.

As was demonstrated in the cases presented, remediation can be very successful but requires dedicated faculty and institutions. Much research has been done on the length of time it takes to remediate a struggling learner. Some research quotes months.[1] One study demonstrated that 15 or more sessions doubled the long-term pass rates at 2 years, compared to less than 10 sessions.[2] Another study showed that remediation decreased the risk of failure to graduate or being placed on probation by approximately 3% per every 1 hour of faculty time spent providing remedial teaching to the learner.[3]

Our understanding of how to successfully remediate struggling learners has grown exponentially in the past 15 years. We now know that it is nearly always possible to turn underperforming learners into competent, safe, and professional practicing colleagues. Engaging in this work will make you a better, more observant teacher of all learners, a more articulate and thoughtful provider of feedback, and a more self-reflective clinician in your own practice. You will become more compassionate of learners who experience the world differently, more informed of the complexities of the evaluative process, and more appreciative of the roles of your deans and program directors. We must never forget that institutions, deans, program directors, and all teaching faculty have societal and ethical obligations to ensure that graduates and colleagues can fulfill their professional roles and responsibilities. Immerse yourself in remediation for the sake of your learners, your overall professional development, and for society at large. ⏻

REFERENCES

1   Zbieranowski I, Takahashi SG, Verma S, Spadafora SM. Remediation of residents in difficulty: a retrospective 10-year review of the experience of a postgraduate board of examiners. *Acad Med.* 2013 Jan 1;88(1):111-6.

2   Winston KA. Core concepts in remediation: lessons learned from a six-year case study. *Med Sci Educ.* 2015;25:307-15.

3   Guerrasio J, Brooks E, Rumack CM, Christensen A, Aagaard EM. Association of characteristics, deficits, and outcomes of residents placed on probation at one institution, 2002-2012. *Acad Med.* 2016 Mar 1;91(3):382-7.

APPENDICES

APPENDIX A Observed Communication Assessment

Date

PA Student

Preceptor/Supervisor

STRONGLY DISAGREE
DISAGREE
NEUTRAL
AGREE
STRONGLY AGREE

BEHAVIOR

○ ○ ○ ○ ○ **Greets patient appropriately**
• smiles, introduces self, shakes hands

○ ○ ○ ○ ○ **Verbally expresses interest in and empathy for patient**
• encouraging statements, reflections, acknowledge patient's feelings, attitudes, beliefs

○ ○ ○ ○ ○ **Nonverbally expresses interest in and empathy for patient**
• allows patient to finish statements
• smiles, eye contact, nods, relaxed/open posture, positioned at patient's eye level

○ ○ ○ ○ ○ **Maintains appropriate demeanor for the visit**
• adjusts mood, tone of voice, facial expressions etc. to fit the patient's needs and the situation
• laughs or uses humor only when appropriate

○ ○ ○ ○ ○ **Uses language patient can understand**
• avoids medical jargon

○ ○ ○ ○ ○ **Encourages questions or feedback from patient**

○ ○ ○ ○ ○ **Closes visit appropriately**
• asks about patient comfort with plan, summarizes the visit, discusses follow-up

○ ○ ○ ○ ○ **Behaves in a mature, appropriate manner** when presenting or discussing patients with other members of the medical team and staff

○ ○ ○ ○ ○ **Interacts in a friendly, courteous manner** with other members of the medical team and staff

COMMENTS:

Example of Clinical Problem-Solving Case

ALIQUOT #1

CC: Altered mental status

HPI: 51-year-old female with no known past medical history was brought into the emergency department by her family for increasing somnolence for the past 3 days. The patient's symptoms began with a headache and mild right upper quadrant abdominal pain several days ago. She then was noted by her family to become more somnolent and unresponsive. In the 24 hours prior to presentation, the patient's altered mental status progressed to the point where she was no longer responding, interacting, or talking with family. Family also noted her to have decreased oral intake and one episode of vomiting. Her family also noted mild yellowing of her eyes.

PMH: None

Medications: Chinese herbal medications (unknown) taken for weight loss

Social History: The patient is housed and lives in San Francisco with her husband and son. She denied ever taking alcohol, tobacco, or drugs. The patient is originally from China but has been in the US for over 10 years.

Family History: Noncontributory

Physical Exam:

Vitals: T 39, BP 98/66, HR 97, RR 12, 100% on room air

General: No apparent distress

HEENT: mildly icteric sclera. Oropharynx clear

CV: Tachycardic, regular, no murmurs, rubs, gallops

Lungs: normal effort, clear to auscultation bilaterally

Abdomen: soft, nondistended, nontender. Trace tenderness to palpation in the RUQ

Neuro: Minimally interactive, does not respond to commands. PERRL, extra-ocular movements intact. No obvious facial asymmetric. Moves all 4 extremities equally and responds to pain equally. Tone within normal limits. Reflexes normal and symmetric.

Given this history and exam, how are you framing this patient's altered mental status? What etiologies are high on your differential diagnosis and why?

APPENDIX B Example of Clinical Problem-Solving Case
(cont'd)

ALIQUOT #2

Labs:

WBC 3.2, Hemoglobin 5.6, Platelets 36

Na 141, K 3.4, Chloride 106, Bicarb 25, BUN 38, Creatinine 1.68,

Glucose 105, Ca 8.3

AST 49, ALT 28, Tbili 2.0

PT 16.3, PTT 35.3, INR 1.4

Lactate 0.8

HIV: negative

Urinalysis: 1+ protein, negative nitrites and leukocyte esterase, 10-20 WBCs, 2-5 RBCs, 2+ amorphous crystals

Utox: positive for benzodiazepines and opiates (both given to patient in emergency department)

Chest X-ray: normal cardiomediastinal silhouette without acute process

CT abdomen/pelvis: normal

CT head: normal

How would you interpret these initial labs and studies? What are you thinking is most likely now on your differential diagnosis?

What further diagnostic tests would you order, and how would you manage this patient if you were admitting her overnight to the hospital?

APPENDIX B Example of Clinical Problem-Solving Case
   (cont'd)

ALIQUOT #3

Further laboratory tests were ordered:

Reticulocyte count 16
LDH 1806
Fibrinogen: 288
Direct coombs test: negative
Haptoglobin <6

How would you interpret these labs? Are there any further studies you would want at this time?

ALIQUOT #4

Further laboratory tests were sent:

MCV – 120
Iron – 84
Ferritin – 1666
Transferrin 180 (ref 180-335)
% saturation 37 (ref 16-60)
B12 level: 119
Methylmalonic Acid: 90 (reference range 0-0.4)
Homocysteine: 117 (reference range <10)
ADAMTS13 level—normal (55%)

What is your final diagnosis to explain this patient's altered mental status? What treatment would you initiate?

APPENDIX C Clinical Reasoning/Case Write-up Feedback Form

Resident Name
_____

Person Filling Out This Form
_____

Date
_____

NOT AT ALL			ALL THE TIME		N/A	HOW WELL DOES THE RESIDENT'S WRITTEN CASE WRITE-UP...
1	2	3	4	5		
○	○	○	○	○	○	**Document a cogent** HPI with all relevant details that is easy to follow and accurate?
○	○	○	○	○	○	**Synthesize all** the salient data, without including or perseverating on irrelevant data in his/her assessment or one-liner?
○	○	○	○	○	○	**Contain comprehensive** and well-prioritized differential diagnoses with a clear, sophisticated discussion of reasoning?
○	○	○	○	○	○	**Demonstrate an excellent** understanding of pathophysiology and medical knowledge?
○	○	○	○	○	○	**Have a complete** problem list and address all concerns/abnormalities on the patient's problem list without missing important details?
○	○	○	○	○	○	**Contain appropriate** management plans based on sound clinical reasoning of the medical team and staff?

What does this resident do well on his/her written case write-ups?

What are areas for growth and further study to improve his/her clinical reasoning and management skills?

Please rate the accuracy of the resident's history and physical examination based on his/her clinical documentation:

○ Struggling/MS3 level   ○ Early Intern Level   ○ Late Intern Level   ○ Resident Level

Please rate the resident's clinical reasoning skills based on his/her clinical documentation:

○ Struggling/MS3 level   ○ Early Intern Level   ○ Late Intern Level   ○ Resident Level

Please rate the resident's ability to comprehensively gather and synthesize clinical data:

○ Struggling/MS3 level   ○ Early Intern Level   ○ Late Intern Level   ○ Resident Level

APPENDIX D Time Management and Organization Resource Sheet

PRE-ROUNDING ON THE WARDS

Pre-rounding should take no more than 2 hours. In those 2 hours you should be able to accomplish the following: (1) get sign-out from back-up, (2) review all vitals, labs, medications, micro, and radiology data, (3) see all your patients, (4) start the majority of your progress notes, and (5) generate a task list/list of to-dos for the day.

The following is an explicit, step-by-step guide to help you accomplish these tasks in the allotted time.

Step 1: Get sign-out from back-up [5 minutes if no drips, 10 min if new drips].

Step 2: Computer time – *this is the only time you should let yourself view a computer during pre-rounding* [25-30 minutes]
- Collect vitals, labs, medications, micro, and radiology results on all your patients. Aim to spend on average 4 minutes reviewing each patient. You can either print out your last progress note or the handoff (both of which will autofill the new vitals and labs for the day) or write the numbers down on the template below.
- If you notice a vital sign or lab value that is abnormal that you would like to discuss in your assessment and plan, circle it and list it as a problem in your A&P later.
- If you are expecting a lab value which is not yet back for a patient, indicate on your task list for you to follow-up that missing lab later in the day.

Step 3: See your patients and decide on your assessment and plan [1.5 hours or about 12 minutes per patient]
- Decide what order you want to see your patients in. Choose an order that both prioritizes seeing sicker patients first and makes geographic sense.
- See and examine the patient. Limit yourself from 3-7 minutes for each patient encounter for patients already on your service previously and

APPENDIX D Time Management and Organization Resource Sheet
   (cont'd)

   10-15 minutes for newly admitted patients that you are less familiar
   with. Seeing different patients will take more or less time depending
   on their complexity.

- After seeing each patient, take 5 minutes to record the following
  sections on your progress note template: subjective, physical exam,
  and your A&P.

- As you are writing your plan, write down action items generated in
  your assessment and plan on your task list. For example, if part of
  your plan is to discontinue IV pain medications, write this on your
  task list.

- *You are not allowed to log into a computer during step 3* unless an urgent
  situation arises, because using a computer will slow you down! All
  computer viewing should be done during Step 2. If a nurse or attending
  pages you to place a non-urgent order, write that reminder down on
  your task list rather than doing it in the moment.

Step 4: Review your task list and triage your tasks.
- Now you have generated your task list for your patients for the day.
- Look at your task list and try to triage what tasks need to be given first
  priority. Highlight those tasks in yellow.
- Putting in time-sensitive orders (like diet orders, antibiotics) and
  calling consults generally need to occur before writing patients for
  labs or discontinuing telemetry.
- If you're having trouble deciding what must be done first, go over
  your task list with your resident and get their input.

APPENDIX D Time Management and Organization Resource Sheet *(cont'd)*

ROUNDING

Spend no more than 3-5 minutes per oral presentation for a patient with only 1-2 active problems and no more than 5-8 minutes for a complex patient. If you're having trouble doing this, ask your resident or attending to time you.

- In general, you should present the "Subjective and Objective" portion of your SOAP note within 2-3 minutes, and your "Assessment and Plan," which you have already thought about and written down while you were pre-rounding, in 2-5 minutes depending on patient complexity.
- If additional to-dos are requested for your patient during rounds (by your attending or resident), write those tasks on your task list while you are rounding on that patient. If you don't write it down, you might forget to do it.

WORKING AFTER ROUNDS

Look at your task list. Highlight tasks that need to occur earlier in the day, such as calling consults, discharging patients, or placing orders that were discussed during rounds. If you are having trouble deciding what tasks need to occur on the early side, go over your task list with your resident for input. Tasks like updating family (unless there is an urgent decision to be made) can happen later in the day.

- As you make your way through each task, darken the box next to the task.
- If one of the tasks is "Order CBC at noon," a helpful organizational tip is to shade in half the box if it is ordered, and shade in the other half once you have followed up the result.

APPENDIX D Time Management and Organization Resource Sheet *(cont'd)*

Name: _____

MRN: _____

Date of Birth: _____

PROGRESS NOTE

Subjective: _____

_____

_____

Objective: _____

Tmax: _____ Tcurent: _____ HR range: _____

BP range: _____ O2 Sat: _____

I/O: _____ Last bowel movement: _____

Physical Exam: _____

_____

_____

_____

Labs/Studies: _____

_____

_____

_____

ASSESSMENT / PLAN: _____

_____

_____

_____

_____

APPENDIX D Time Management and Organization Resource Sheet *(cont'd)*

TASK LIST

Patient Name

☐ _____   ☐ _____
☐ _____   ☐ _____
☐ _____   ☐ _____
☐ _____   ☐ _____
☐ _____   ☐ _____
☐ _____   ☐ _____
☐ _____   ☐ _____

Patient Name

☐ _____   ☐ _____
☐ _____   ☐ _____
☐ _____   ☐ _____
☐ _____   ☐ _____
☐ _____   ☐ _____
☐ _____   ☐ _____
☐ _____   ☐ _____

Patient Name

☐ _____   ☐ _____
☐ _____   ☐ _____
☐ _____   ☐ _____
☐ _____   ☐ _____
☐ _____   ☐ _____
☐ _____   ☐ _____
☐ _____   ☐ _____

APPENDIX E Oral Presentation Feedback Form (1/3)

Resident Name
_____

Attending Name
_____

Date
_____

1	2	3	4	5	HOW OFTEN DID THE RESIDENT...
○	○	○	○	○	**Present** information in the expected order?
○	○	○	○	○	**Adhere** to a reasonable time frame (~10 minutes)?
○	○	○	○	○	**Have a complete** problem list during A&P?
○	○	○	○	○	**Integrate** new data into the problem list (e.g., discussing a new fever or a new abnormal lab)?
○	○	○	○	○	**Re-prioritize** the problem list to reflect acuity/importance of problems?
○	○	○	○	○	**Have a well-thought-out** differential diagnosis and assessment for each important problem?
○	○	○	○	○	**Editorialize** or provide opinions prior to the A&P?
○	○	○	○	○	**Fail to present** important data prior to the A&P?
○	○	○	○	○	**Spend too much** time presenting unimportant data?

(Scale: 1 = NONE OF THE TIME, 5 = ALL OF THE TIME)

What does the learner do well on his/her oral presentations? [List 3 examples]

What does the learner need to work on with his/her oral presentations? [List 1 or 2 examples]

APPENDIX E Oral Presentation Feedback Form (2/3)

Please rate the resident's oral presentation skills on the following scale from 1–5 using the following criteria.

○ 1 Deficient	○ 2 Direct Supervision	○ 3 Indirect Supervision	○ 4 Unsupervised Practice	○ 5 Aspirational
Presentation too long (>12 minutes), disorganized and missing important data	Presentation organized, contain all the essential data, may include some non-essential data	Presentation 10 minutes, long, organized, and contains all essential data	Presentation 10 minutes or less, organized, and contains all essential data	Presentation under 10 minutes, organized, and contains all essential information
Important information missing from presentations	Information presented in the appropriate order	Information presented in the appropriate order	Information presented in the appropriate order	Information presented in the appropriate order
Assessment and plan does not address crucial problems pertaining to patient	Problem list contains new developments in patient care (e.g., if a patient is hypertensive) with a good clinical assessment	Problem list complete, contains new developments in patient care, and prioritized to contain the most crucial problems first	Problem list complete, contains new developments in patient care, and prioritized to contain the most crucial problems first	Problem list complete, prioritized, and contains new developments in patient care
Lacking an organized clinical assessment	Clinical assessments may require supervisor input	Differential diagnoses for all problems, management plans are rudimentary	Differential diagnoses for all problems are complete, well-considered, and management plans are reasonable and complete	Differential diagnoses for all problems are complete, well-considered and management plans are reasonable, complete, and demonstrate considerable critical thinking, risk/benefit analyses, and take into account patient preferences if appropriate
Differential diagnoses are complete	Differential diagnoses capture 3-4 diagnoses but miss important diagnoses			

195

APPENDIX E Oral Presentation Feedback Form (3/3)

ADDITIONAL NOTES/COMMENTS (OPTIONAL):

Signature of Evaluator:

Date you discussed this evaluation with the resident:

GLOSSARY

academic success center – Some institutions combine all their student resources into one department – including disabilities support, tutors, mental health services, remediation, etc. This is one example of what to call such a department. Other examples are listed in the glossary as well.

Accreditation Council for Graduate Medical Education (ACGME) competencies

- **Medical Knowledge** – Demonstrate knowledge about established and evolving biomedical, clinical, and cognate (e.g. epidemiological and social-behavioral) sciences and the application of this knowledge to patient care
- **Patient Care** – Employ care that is compassionate, appropriate, and effective for the treatment of health problems and the promotion of health
- **Interpersonal Skills and Communication** – Demonstrate effective information exchange and teaming with patients, patients' families, and professional associates
- **Professionalism** – Embrace a commitment to carrying out professional responsibilities, adherence to ethical principles, and sensitivity to a diverse patient population
- **Problem-Based Learning and Improvement** – Investigate and evaluate one's own patient care practices, appraise and assimilate scientific evidence, and improve patient care practices, including being receptive to and incorporating feedback
- **Systems-Based Practice** – Demonstrate an awareness of and responsiveness to the larger context and system of health care, as well as the ability to call effectively on other resources in the system to provide optimal health care

Board Vitals® Exam – A company that provides practice board exam questions and practice exams. While as helpful for remediation as they are great for foundation building, the editor found them insufficiently challenging for final board studying in the subjects that she reviewed, as the questions and content were more foundational and often 1-step questions.

centralized remediation – Remediation that is performed by a small team of experts or developing experts for several academic branches, such as all students, multiple residency programs, all graduate medical education or the entire campus

chief resident – A resident who is in their final year of residency or who is completing an additional year of residency and who has been acknowledged as a leader among their peers. Chief residents are often entrusted with teaching and assisting with assessments, evaluation, and remediation of junior learners.

clinical competency committee (CCC) – A requirement of the ACGME, it is a residency-level committee that participates in the assessment and evaluation of its residents.

clinical reasoning – The ability to apply one's knowledge to the clinical problem or chief complaint and data as presented by the patient case

clinical skills – Skills requiring manual dexterity, such as the physical exam and procedural skills

Clinical Skills Verification – An exam established by the American Board of Psychiatry and Neurology to be administered by residency training programs. It includes a directed observed assessment of a resident's physician-patient relationship, a psychiatric interview including the mental status exam and a case presentation.

compliance officer – A hospital employee tasked with ensuring that institutional policies and rules are being followed

corrective action plan – One of many names used for a remediation plan; also called an individualized learning plan

counseling center – Provides mental health services such as therapy and medication management. Other examples of what to call such a department are listed in the glossary as well.

deliberate practice – Purposeful and systematic practice incorporating focused attention on practice after receiving feedback, reflecting on that feedback, and altering one's practice with the goal of improved performance

departmental chair – An individual who leads and oversee the research, clinical, and education endeavors of a medical department (e.g. general surgery, medicine)

designated institutional officer (DIO) – An individual who is designated with the authority and responsibility to oversee all of the residency (and fellowship) training programs at their institution. The DIO is responsible for assuring that the individual training programs meet the ACGME requirements.

director of clinical training – Similar to an attending physician in the United States, it is the medical specialist working with the resident team and teaching staff.

director of clinical education – Referenced in Case Study #1, a physician assistant case, this position is similar to the dean of student clerkships, for which the director of clinical education oversees clinical rotations, instruction, assessment methods, evaluations, curriculum coordination, and successful achievement of learner competence.

employee assistance program (EAP) –A voluntary, work-based program that offers free and confidential assessments, short-term counseling, referrals, and follow-up services to employees who have personal and/or work-related problems

entrustable professional activities – A key task of a medical specialty that an individual can be trusted to perform

feeding forward, also known as learner handoffs or learner handovers – Passing information about a learner from one supervisor or faculty member to another within or across multiple rotations or academic years

FERPA (The Family Education Rights and Privacy Act) – A federal law passed in the United States to protect the privacy of student education records. There are many misconceptions about this law which harm students. Please discuss your concerns with legal counsel or review the law which is available online through the US Department of Education.

fitness for duty, also known as fitness to care – The minimum acceptable standards of physical and mental health that a learner must possess to ensure their fitness to care for patients safely

fixed mindset – Existing on a continuum with growth mindset, fixed mindset can be thought of in the context of resiliency and the ability to persevere through educational challenges. People with a fixed mindset see their own mistakes, challenges, and setback as signs of stupidity and incompetence and are quicker to give up.

graduate medical education committee – The institutional policy-setting body which monitors the activity of all residency programs. It includes resident members.

growth mindset – Existing on a continuum with fixed mindset, growth mindset can be thought of in the context of resiliency and the ability to persevere through educational challenges. People with growth mindset see their own mistakes, challenges and setbacks as opportunities to learn and become better clinicians.

HIPAA (Health Insurance Portability and Accountability Act) – Per the CDC, a federal law that required the creation of national standards to protect sensitive patient health information from being disclosed without the patient's consent or knowledge. Like FERPA, there are many misconceptions about this law which harm patients. Please discuss your concerns with legal counsel or review the law which is available online through the Department of Health and Human Services.

house medical officer – Following medical school, this position is similar to a transitional year of residency in the United States. The training is comprised of rotations in general medicine, surgery and emergency medicine, and other general medical specialties.

house staff – Resident and fellow physicians

illness script – An organized mental summary of a clinician's knowledge of a disease

international medical graduate – Residents who received their medical school training in a country other than where they are completing their residency training

The Match – A process through which fourth-year medical students apply, interview, and are paired with their future residency programs

medical education unit – Similar to a team of residents, fellows, and teaching staff in the United States

mental well-being – Any stressor that the learner brings into the learning environment that affects their ability to learn, such as depression, anxiety, substance abuse, a learning disorder, birth of a child, sick parent, etc.

mini-clinical examination – A 10- to 20-minute direct observation assessment of a learner-patient interaction to facilitate formative assessment of core clinical skills

observed structured clinical encounter – A multi-case or patient clinical skills assessment method that is based on objective testing and direct observation of learner performance. It is designed to test real-world competence.

observed structured teaching encounter – A multi-case or learner teaching skills assessment method that is based on objective testing and direct observation of teacher performance. It is designed to test real-world competence.

office of case management services – Serves as an advocate and guide to the student towards additional resources and services the learners may need (e.g., mental health services, office of disability and resource services, healthcare services, etc.) Other examples of what to name such a department are listed in the glossary as well.

PACKRAT (physician assistant clinical knowledge rating and assessment tool) – A national formative comprehensive written assessment given periodically in PA school to assess student progress. Given as a multiple-choice question test.

probation – Often (but not always) the result of failing grades, it is intended to serve as a red flag to the learner of their need to change their academic trajectory. Since probation is also reportable beyond training, it also serves as a red flag that the learner may need extra monitoring post-graduation.

program director – An individual who is in charge of leading, developing, and improving the educational experience of a group of residents or fellows and is responsible for determining their competence for graduation

program evaluation committee (PEC) – Another name for a committee that serves a function similar to the clinical competency committee (CCC)

red flags – Warning signs of future poor performance such as previous poor exam scores, low grades on clinical rotations, and prior probationary status

RIME – Developed by Lou Pangaro, a system for categorizing the stages of clinical reasoning development: reporter, interpreter, manager, educator

schema – A cognitive tool that allows clinicians to systematically approach a clinical problem by providing an organizing scaffold

The Scramble (now called "The SOAP" which stands for Supplemental Offer and Acceptance Program) – the process following The Match, which provides an opportunity for medical students who did not get into a residency program to secure a residency position from the remaining positions available

SOAP note – A method of documentation employed by clinicians that is divided into 4 sections: subjective, objective, assessment, and plan.

standardized or simulated cases – Each patient or professional represents the same patient case in the same way every time

student services – Some institutions combine all student resources into one department, including disabilities support, tutors, mental health services, remediation, etc. Other examples of what to call such a department are listed in the glossary as well.

System 1 thinking – Implicit, automatic, pattern recognition decision making or nonanalytical reasoning

System 2 thinking – Explicit, controlled, rational, effortful, relatively slow analytical reasoning

time management and organization – The ability to stay focused on different tasks and to use one's time and energy effectively and efficiently to complete necessary tasks

underrepresented minorities (URMs) – Defined by the Association of American Medical Colleges (AAMC) as racial and ethnic populations that are under-represented in the medical profession relative to their numbers in the general population. Similar struggles may be seen by other minorities such as first-generation college students, rural students, lower socioeconomic students, etc.

ABOUT THE AUTHOR

Jeannette Guerrasio, MD

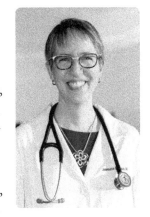

For over a decade, Jeannette Guerrasio, MD, practiced internal medicine as a hospitalist when she was a professor of medicine at the University of Colorado School of Medicine. In 2019, she transitioned her career to primary care.

While at the University of Colorado, Dr. Guerrasio dedicated her academic career to working with struggling medical learners. She has worked one-on-one with almost 1,000 struggling medical students, residents, fellows, and faculty, as well as nurse practitioner, physician assistant, physical therapy, and optometry students.

At the University of Colorado, Dr. Guerrasio built a unique and highly successful remediation program which includes the development of individualized learning plans. She has provided institution-level faculty development workshops and has lectured and led workshops at regional, national, and international conferences, giving her a national and international reputation for her work and expertise in this area. From these experiences she wrote a very successful book, *Remediation of the Struggling Medical Learner*, now in its second edition.

Dr. Guerrasio has won numerous awards for her teaching, mentoring, and humanism. She was honored with the National Society of General Internal

Medicine Scholarship in Medical Education Award and the Association of American Medical Colleges Southern Group on Educational Affairs Medical Education Scholarship Award. She was inducted into the Academy of Medical Educators in 2012, and into the University of Colorado's President's Teaching Scholars Guild in 2016. In 2019, she was awarded the John C. Leonard Award from the Association of Hospital Medical Education.

In 2021, Dr. Guerrasio founded Medicine Within Reach, PLLC, to bridge her many teaching endeavors, all of which aim to make medicine accessible to everyone, including students and patients. Using her unique ability to make complex concepts easy to understand and less intimidating, she now also writes for the general public.

Additional information about
the author and upcoming events are available at
www.medicinewithinreach.us

ABOUT THE ASSOCIATION FOR

HOSPITAL MEDICAL EDUCATION

(AHME)

The Association for Hospital Medical Education, founded in 1956, is a national, non-profit organization involved in the continuum of hospital-based medical education. AHME's members represent several hundred teaching hospitals, academic medical centers, and consortia which are involved in the delivery of undergraduate, graduate, and continuing medical education. The mission of AHME is to promote improvement in medical education to meet health care needs, serve as a forum and resource for medical education information, develop professionals in the field of medical education, and advocate the value of medical education in health care.

To fulfill its mission, the Association annually provides a three-day educational conference (AHME Institute), one-day educational sessions (AHME Academy), and a series of six webinars. AHME publishes the *Guide to Medical Education in the Teaching Hospital* (a practical resource for medical education professionals), *Remediation of the Struggling Medical Learner* (a structured approach to identifying and supporting residents and students who aren't progressing at an expected pace), *Remediation Case Studies: Helping Struggling Medical Learners*, and two issues of *AHME News* annually. Additional resources are also made available on the AHME website (www.ahme.org). AHME has secured external funding to support clinical performance-improvement activities, solicited and reviewed proposals from member institutions, and awarded grants to support these projects. AHME also publishes the *Journal for Continuing Education in the Health Professions*, a peer-reviewed publication, in collaboration with the Alliance for Continuing Education in the Health Professions (ACEHP) and the Society of Academic Continuing Medical Education (SACME).

AHME supports four interest groups, which include the Council of Institutional Leaders, the Council of Program Administrators and Coordinators, the Council on Professional and Faculty Development, and the Council of Transitional Year Program Directors. The Association is a member organization of the Accreditation Council for Continuing Medical Education, an associate member organization of the Council of Medical Specialty Societies, as well as a liaison organization of the National Resident Matching Program. It also enjoys collaborative relationships with a number of other accreditation, regulatory, and professional organizations with an interest in medical education.

INDEX

The letter *t* following a page number denotes a table.
The letter *a* following a page number denotes an appendix.
The letter *f* following a page number denotes a figure.

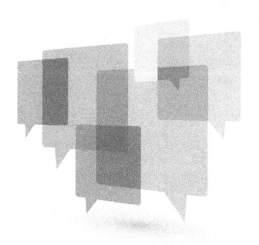

CPSIA information can be obtained
at www.ICGtesting.com
Printed in the USA
BVHW060825281221
625045BV00018B/573